Basic Notes in Psychiatry

Fourth Edition

Dr Michael I Levi MB BS MRCPsych
Consultant Psychiatrist
Bradford District Care Trust
Horton Park Centre
Bradford, West Yorkshire, UK

Radcliffe Publishing
Oxford • Seattle

Radcliffe Publishing Ltd
18 Marcham Road
Abingdon
Oxon OX14 1AA
United Kingdom

www.radcliffe-oxford.com
Electronic catalogue and worldwide online ordering facility.

First edition 1989 (published by Kluwer Academic Publishers)
Second edition 1998 (published by Petroc Press)
Third edition 2003 (published by Petroc Press)

The views expressed in this book reflect the experience of the author. Any
products referred to by the author should only be used as recommended in the
manufacturers' data sheets or summaries of product characteristics (SPCs).

British Library Cataloguing in Publication Data

A catalogue record for this book is available from the British Library.

ISBN 1 85775 716 5

Typeset by Advance Typesetting Ltd, Oxford
Printed and bound by TJ International Ltd, Padstow, Cornwall

Contents

Foreword to fourth edition

There are a great many books and journal papers that the stressed candidate will be required to read and understand before, at last, going forward into that ultimate rite of passage, namely the Membership Examination of the Royal College of Psychiatrists. Now all your exhausting revision work has been finally completed, I commend you to this latest version of Mike Levi's excellent revision guide. It concisely covers all the key points you will need to cover the Part 2 exam syllabus.

This fourth edition of Mike's popular book is once again a vital revision aid which will remind you of all you have already learned, and will help you put all this information into a logical order. It should help to ease your passage through the examination and give you a smooth landing on the other side.

It has helped a great many of your colleagues who have gone before, and I hope it will do the same for you – the best of luck.

Simon Baugh
Medical Director
Bradford District NHS Care Trust
West Yorkshire
August 2005

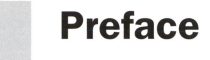

Preface

Following the popularity of the third edition, I was encouraged to write this edition for junior hospital psychiatrists, general practitioners and medical students.

I have completely updated the management sections of each chapter, where appropriate, in the light of current knowledge. I have also revised the diagnostic terms used throughout the book, where appropriate, with the advent of new systems of classification since the appearance of the first edition in 1989.

Michael I Levi
August 2005

Introduction

The purpose of writing this book is to provide a concise summary of general adult psychiatry in the form of notes. I have based these notes on what is generally regarded to be the most comprehensive textbook[1] for the MRCPsych examination. These notes represent my own view of current clinical practice.

The book is intended to have a wide readership – particularly among junior hospital psychiatrists, general practitioners and medical students. In addition, it will also be useful to psychiatric nurses, psychiatric social workers and clinical psychologists.

Reference

1 Gelder M, Lopez-Ibor JJ and Andreasen N (eds) (2003) *New Oxford Textbook of Psychiatry*. Oxford University Press, Oxford.

CHAPTER 1

The history, mental state examination and formulation

As in any branch of medicine, psychiatry begins with taking a good history and examining the patient. The history is very similar in format to that taken in general medicine, while the mental state examination is something very particular to psychiatry. Having done both of these, it is then necessary to provide a formulation – i.e. a summary of the case presented in an integrated or synthesised fashion. This chapter deals with, in turn, the history, the mental state examination and the formulation.

The history

Age/Marital Status/Occupation

Source of referral

1 PC/HPC (presenting complaint/history of the presenting complaint): Principal symptoms or complaints and their duration; associated disturbance in appetite, weight, sleep and sexual drive; effects on patient's ability to cope socially or with work.
2 PPH (past psychiatric history): Previous hospital admissions with psychiatric illness. Treatment given. How well did patient remain in between admissions?
3 PMH/PSH (past medical history/past surgical history): Previous hospital admissions with physical illness or for operations.
4 FH (family history):
    (a) **Mother and father** – current age or, if dead, age at death and cause of death; occupations.
    (b) **Sisters and brothers** – names, ages, marital status, occupation.

(c) **FPH** (family psychiatric history) – history of any psychiatric illness in the family.

(d) **FMH** (family medical history) – history of any physical illness in the family.

(e) **Current relationships** – with parents, siblings and other relatives.

5 PH (personal history) – born and bred:

(a) **Birth** – any prematurity or low birth weight; any difficulties during delivery.

(b) **Pre-school development** – any delay in achieving milestones; any separation from parents; relationships with parents, siblings, other children and adults at this age.

(c) **School** – age of starting and finishing school; type of school attended; academic qualifications; relationships with pupils and teachers.

(d) **Occupations** – chronological list of jobs; if multiple changes, enquire about the reasons; relationships with workmates and superiors.

(e) **Psychosexual history** – age of onset of puberty; first steady relationship; first sexual intercourse; any evidence of physical, sexual or emotional abuse; if married, age at marriage and age of spouse at marriage; any psychiatric or physical illness in spouse; relationship with spouse; if children, give chronological list of their names, age and sex; any psychiatric or physical illness in children; relationship with children.

6 **Smoke** – current and past smoking habits.

7 **Drink** – current and past drinking habits.

8 **Drugs** – drugs, medicines or tablets patient is currently taking; any abuse of illicit drugs (e.g. cannabis, amphetamines, opiates).

9 **Allergies** – any known allergies.

10 **Social circumstances** – current type of residence (e.g. flat, house); composition of household.

11 **Forensic history** – any trouble with the law or police; any convictions.

12 **PMP** (premorbid personality) – the patient's personality before first admission to hospital with psychiatric illness:

(a) **Relationships** – few friends or many.

(b) **Character** – outgoing or reserved.

(c) **Mood** – cheerful or gloomy; steady or changeable.

(d) **Leisure activities** – preference for company or solitude.

The mental state examination

1 **Appearance and behaviour:**

(a) **Dress and self-care** – tidy or dishevelled, well-groomed or unkempt; describe actual clothes.

   (b) **Manner** – hostile or helpful, aggressive or amiable.
   (c) **Posture and movement** – tense or relaxed, overactive or slowed-up.
   (d) **Appropriateness** – in touch with surroundings or listening to hallucinatory voices.
2 **Speech** – pressure or poverty of speech; spontaneous or hesitant; coherent or incoherent; neologisms.
3 **Mood:**
   (a) Subjective report.
   (b) Depression or elation.
   (c) Anxiety, irritability, fear or hostility.
   (d) Incongruity or blunting of affect.
   (e) Suicidal ideation. Homicidal ideation.
4 **Thought:**
   (a) Content – worries or preoccupations; obsessions or delusions; passivity phenomena; persecutory ideation.
   (b) Form – pressure or poverty of thought; thought blocking; loosening of associations or flight of ideas or perseveration; interpretation of proverbs.
5 **Perception** – hallucinations; illusions; depersonalisation or derealisation.
6 **Cognition:**
   (a) **Orientation** – in time, place, person and age.
   (b) **Attention and concentration** – subjective report, days of week backwards (DOWB) or months of year backwards (MOYB); serial sevens test or serial threes test; digit span forwards and backwards (five to seven numbers).
   (c) **Memory** – subjective report and:
      (i) **Immediate memory** – name and address, immediate recall; Babcock sentence; digit span (as above).
      (ii) **Recent memory** – name and address, five-minute recall; menu of most recent meal.
      (iii) **Remote memory** – personal events recalled from several years ago; assessed in the history.
   (d) **Grasp** – Prime Minister of UK; President of USA; reigning monarch of UK; any item of current affairs.
7 **Insight:**
   (a) Does the patient consider himself ill in psychological terms?
   (b) Does the patient feel in need of treatment?

The formulation

1 **Introduction** – salient features of history (positives and negatives).

2   **Current mental state examination** – label psychopathological features.
3   **Diagnosis** – support with reasons from mental state examination and history.
4   **Differential diagnosis:**
   (a)   The diagnostic hierarchy is useful in deciding this:
      (i)   Personality disorders.
      (ii)   Anxiety disorders.
      (iii)   Delusional disorders.
      (iv)   Affective disorders.
      (v)   Schizophrenia.
      (vi)   Organic disorders.
   A high-priority condition (e.g. organic disorders) can be accompanied by the symptoms of a low-priority condition (e.g. anxiety disorders), but only the high-priority condition need be diagnosed.
   (b)   There should be a maximum of two conditions to be considered in the differential diagnosis – to indicate you have synthesised the case.
   (c)   Each condition should be supported with reasons from the mental state examination and history.
5   **Aetiology:**
   (a)   Predisposing factors:
      (i)   FPH.
      (ii)   PMP.
      (iii)   Parental separation/loss.
      (iv)   Relationship difficulties with parents.
      (v)   Childhood abuse.
      (vi)   Adverse social circumstances.
   (b)   Precipitating factors:
      (i)   Iatrogenic.
      (ii)   Non-compliance with medication.
      (iii)   Stressors, e.g. work pressure.
      (iv)   High expressed emotion (high 'EE').
      (v)   Alcohol abuse.
      (vi)   Illicit drug abuse.
      (vii)   Post-operative.
      (viii) Post-partum.
      (ix)   Acute relapse of medical condition.
   (c)   Maintaining factors:
      (i)   Poor or non-compliance with psychotropic medication.
      (ii)   Ongoing substance abuse.
      (iii)   Chronic medical condition.
      (iv)   Ongoing relationship difficulties.
      (v)   Unresolved grief.
      (vi)   Ongoing social/financial problems.

6   Investigations:
   (a) More information: Speak to informants (e.g. spouse, relatives, friends); speak to general practitioner; obtain reports from other agencies (e.g. school, employers); old case notes.
   (b) Further assessments:
       (i)   **Physical** – full physical examination, blood tests, urine tests, X-rays, EEG (electroencephalogram), ECG (electrocardiogram).
       (ii)   **Social** – social worker's report; family interview.
       (iii) **Psychological** – psychometry (i.e. assessment of general intelligence, personality and neuropsychological status by a clinical psychologist).
       (iv)   **Others** – observations by nursing staff; occupational therapy assessments (e.g. assessment of daily living).

7   Management:
   (a) Short term: In-patient versus out-patient; compulsory order; immediate physical treatment; contributions by nursing staff, social worker and occupational therapist.
   (b) Long term:
       (i)   **Physical** – subsequent physical treatment with drugs and ECT (electroconvulsive therapy).
       (ii)   **Social** – part played by other members of the multidisciplinary team (e.g. social worker, community psychiatric nurse); social provisions or supports; family involvement; rehabilitation.
       (iii) **Psychological** – supportive psychotherapy versus formal psychotherapy versus brief interviews to assess progress; behavioural therapy (relaxation training and anxiety management training); cognitive therapy.

8   Prognosis:
   (a) State whether poor or good with reasons, e.g. good prognosis because of acute onset and presence of a precipitating factor.
   (b) Consider the prognosis both for this episode and in the long term.

CHAPTER 2

The symptoms and signs of mental illness

As in any branch of medicine, making a diagnosis in psychiatry is based on:

1 **Eliciting the symptoms** – by asking the patient about the presenting complaint and the history of the presenting complaint.
2 **Eliciting the signs** – by examining the mental state of the patient for psychopathological features.

The framework for eliciting the symptoms and signs is the history and mental state examination, as detailed in Chapter 1. The purpose of this chapter is to describe the various psychopathological features which may be seen in the mental state examination. The diagnostic significance of each feature will be pointed out in the various chapters to follow on general adult psychiatry.

I   APPEARANCE AND BEHAVIOUR

1 **Appearance** – mood may be expressed in the form of:
   (a) **Appearance** – facial expression, posture.
   (b) **Manner** – response to others.
   (c) **Motility** – degree and form of movements.
2 **Behaviour** – there are several motor disorders of general behaviour:
   (a) **Echolalia** – repetition by the patient of the interviewer's words or phrases.
   (b) **Echopraxia** – imitation by the patient of the interviewer's movements.
   (c) **Stereotypy** – regular, repetitive non goal-directed movement (i.e. purposeless).
   (d) **Mannerism** – abnormal, repetitive goal-directed movement (i.e. of some functional significance).
   (e) **Chorea** – random, jerky movements, resembling fragments of goal-directed behaviour (i.e. semi-purposeful).
   (f) **Athetosis** – slow, writhing, semi-rotatory movements.
   (g) **Waxy flexibility** – the patient's limb can be placed in an awkward posture and remain fixed in position over a long period, despite asking the patient to relax (also called catalepsy).

(h) **Mitmachen** – the patient's body can be placed in any posture, despite asking the patient to resist all movements. When released, the patient returns to the resting position (cf. waxy flexibility).

(i) **Mitgehen** – an extreme form of mitmachen in which the patient will move in any direction with very slight pressure.

(j) **Gegenhalten (opposition)** – the patient will oppose attempts at passive movement with a force equal to that being applied (cf. mitmachen).

(k) **Negativism** – an extreme form of gegenhalten, in which there is an apparently motiveless resistance to suggestion or attempts at movement.

(l) **Automatic obedience** – the patient does whatever the interviewer asks of him irrespective of the consequences.

(m) **Ambitendence** – the patient begins to make a movement but, before completing it, starts the opposite movement.

(n) **Stupor** – a state of more or less complete loss of activity with no reaction to external stimuli, although the patient is conscious.

(o) **Perseveration** – the senseless repetition of a previously requested movement, i.e. the repetition of a motor response after the stimulus is withdrawn.

II **SPEECH**

1 **Pressure of speech** – rapid and copious speech, as thoughts crowd into the patient's mind in quick succession.

2 **Poverty of speech** – slow and sparse speech, as thoughts enter the patient's mind only occasionally.

3 **Neologisms** – the patient uses words or phrases invented by himself.

4 **Mutism** – the total loss of speech.

III **MOOD**

1 **Incongruity of affect (inappropriate affect)** – the mood is not in keeping with the mood that would ordinarily be expected, e.g. the patient may laugh when told about a bereavement.

2 **Blunting of affect (flattening of affect)** – sustained emotional indifference or diminution of emotional response.

NB: *Mood and affect are often used interchangeably to mean the same thing. Technically, however, there is a difference between them:*
– *Affect – a short-lived emotion.*
– *Mood – a sustained emotion.*

IV **THOUGHT**

1 **Content:**

(a) **Obsessions** – recurrent, persistent thoughts, impulses, or images that the patient regards as absurd and alien, while recognising them as the product of his own mind. Attempts are made (at least early on) to resist or ignore them. Frequently the obsessions are of an aggressive or sexual nature.

(b) **Delusion** – a false belief with the following characteristics: firmly held despite evidence to the contrary; out of keeping with the person's educational and cultural background; content often bizarre; often infused with a sense of great personal meaning.

(c) **Passivity phenomena** – the individual experiences interference with, or outside control of, his thinking, feeling, perception or behaviour. This is due to the apparent disintegration of boundaries between the self and the surrounding world. There are several types:

(i) **Thought insertion** – the experience of thoughts being put into the mind by some external force.

(ii) **Thought withdrawal** – the experience of thoughts being taken out of the mind by some external force.

(iii) **Thought broadcasting** – the experience that others can 'read' the individual's thoughts as they are 'broadcast' from his mind.

(iv) **'Made' volition** – the experience that free will is removed and behaviour is controlled by some external force.

NB: *Technically passivity phenomena are disorders of the possession of thought. However, by convention they are included under disorders of the content of thought:*

2 **Form:**

(a) **Pressure of thought** – ideas arise in unusual variety and abundance, and pass through the mind rapidly.

(b) **Poverty of thought** – the patient has only a few ideas, which lack variety and abundance, and pass through the mind slowly.

(c) **Thought blocking** – the experience of the patient's mind going entirely blank in the middle of a train of thought.

(d) **Loosening of associations** – loss of the normal structure of thinking. Muddled and illogical conversations that cannot be clarified by further enquiry. It can take several forms:

(i) **Knight's move (derailment)** – a transition from one topic to another with no logical relationship between the two topics and no evidence of links between these topics as seen in flight of ideas (*see* below).

(ii) **Word salad (verbigeration)** – disruption of both the connection between topics and the finer grammatical structure of speech.

(iii) **Talking past the point (vorbeireden)** – the patient seems always about to get near to the matter in hand, but never quite reaches it.

(e) **Flight of ideas** – the patient's thoughts and conversation move quickly from one topic to another, so that one train of thought is not completed before another appears. The links between these rapidly changing topics are understandable, because they occur in normal thinking, i.e. rhyming, punning, clang associations and responding to distracting cues in the immediate surroundings.

(f) **Perseveration** – the persistent and inappropriate repetition of the same thoughts. In response to a series of different questions the patient gives the correct answer to the first, but continues to answer subsequent questions with the answer to the first question.

NB: Technically pressure of thought, poverty of thought and thought blocking are disorders of the stream of thought. However, by convention they are included under disorders of the form of thought.

V PERCEPTION

1 **Hallucinations** – perceptions which arise in the absence of any external stimulus.

2 **Illusions** – distortions of perceptions of real objects.

3 **Depersonalisation** – a change in self-awareness such that the person feels unreal.

4 **Derealisation** – a change in self-awareness such that the environment feels unreal.

VI COGNITION

1 **Age disorientation** – the patient can correctly give his date of birth and the current date, but gives a gross underestimate of his current age.

2 **Serial sevens test** – subtraction of serial sevens from 100.

3 **Serial threes test** – subtraction of serial threes from 40.

4 **Digit span** – a series of digits repeated forwards and backwards. Begin with five numbers and build up to seven.

5 **Babcock sentence** – the patient can correctly repeat the sentence: 'one thing a nation must have to become rich and great is a large secure supply of wood'.

CHAPTER 3

Personality disorders

Definition

Deeply ingrained, maladaptive patterns of behaviour; recognisable in adolescence or earlier; continuing throughout most of adult life; either the patient or others have to suffer; there is an adverse effect on the individual or society.

Epidemiology

More commonly diagnosed in:
1 age group 18–35
2 male sex
3 lower social class.

Clinical features

I   **Affective personality disorder** – three groups:
1 **Depressive personality disorder** – always low in spirits; persistently gloomy view of life; brood about misfortunes; worry unduly; strong sense of duty; little capacity for enjoyment.
2 **Hyperthymic personality disorder** – habitually cheerful and optimistic; striking zest for living; poor judgement; periods of irritability when aims frustrated.
3 **Cyclothymic personality disorder** – alternate between being low in spirits and being cheerful and optimistic; gloomy defeatist approach to life as mood changes from hyperthymic to depressive; reduced energy.

II   **Anankastic personality disorder** (obsessional personality disorder) – lack of adaptability to new situations; high moral standards; humourless approach to life; miserly; sensitivity to criticism; indecision; emotionally constricted.

III   **Antisocial personality disorder** (sociopathic or asocial personality disorder) – impulsive actions; lack of guilt; failure to make loving relationships; failure to learn from adverse experiences.

IV   **Asthenic personality disorder** (passive or dependent personality disorder) – weak-willed; unduly compliant; lack vigour; lack self-reliance; avoid responsibility; little capacity for enjoyment.

V   **Avoidant personality disorder** – hypersensitive to rejection; low self-esteem; unwillingness to enter into relationships; desire for acceptance.

VI   **Borderline personality disorder** – unstable relationships; undue anger; variable moods; chronic boredom; doubts about personal identity; intolerance of being left alone; self-injury; impulsive behaviour that is damaging to the person.

VII   **Explosive personality disorder** – instability of mood with outbursts of anger and violence; no other difficulties in relationships (cf. antisocial personality disorder).

VIII **Histrionic personality disorder** – self-dramatisation; a self-centred approach to personal relationships; a craving for excitement and novelty.

IX   **Narcissistic personality disorder** – grandiose sense of self-importance; preoccupation with fantasies of unlimited success, power and intellectual brilliance; attention demanding but show little warm feeling in return; exploitative but do not give favours in return.

X   **Paranoid personality disorder** – strong sense of self-importance; suspicious; hypersensitive; cold affect; argumentative and stubborn.

XI   **Passive–aggressive personality disorder** – passive resistance to demands for adequate performance; stubborn; intentionally inefficient.

XII   **Schizoid personality disorder** – introspective; prone to engage in an inner world of fantasy rather than take action; lack of emotional warmth and rapport; self-sufficient and detached; aloof and humourless; incapable of expressing tenderness or affection; shy; often eccentric; insensitive; ill-at-ease in company.

XIII **Schizotypal personality disorder** – superstitious ideas; an interest in telepathy and clairvoyance; unrealistic (magical) thinking; odd forms of speech.

Aetiology

I   **Genetic** – no satisfactory evidence about the genetic contribution to personality disorders.
II **Body build (Kretschmer):**
  1 Pyknic (stocky and rounded) build – related to cyclothymic personality disorder.
  2 Asthenic (lean and narrow) build – related to schizoid personality disorder.
III **Psychoanalytic theory** – serious difficulty in passing through the anal stage of development will result in anankastic personality disorder.
IV **Childhood influences on personality development** – maternal separation has been proposed as a cause of antisocial personality disorder.

Differential diagnosis

I   **Exclude any organic disorders** – e.g. focal or diffuse organic brain disease, epilepsy, alcohol or drug abuse.
II **Exclude any functional psychiatric illness** – e.g. schizophrenia, affective disorders, neurotic disorders.

Management

I   **Physical:**
  1 **Short term** – anxiolytic drugs or neuroleptics may be given for short periods at times of unusual stress.
  2 **Long term** – neuroleptics may be helpful in paranoid and schizotypal personality disorders.
II **Social** – supervision and support are often beneficial. This can be given by a doctor, social worker or psychiatric nurse.
III **Psychological:**
  1 For the majority, psychotherapy is not indicated. Group psychotherapy is more helpful than individual psychotherapy. Confrontative psychotherapy is more helpful than interpretative psychotherapy. Psychotherapy is least likely to help people with antisocial personality disorders, although some are helped by large group psychotherapy in the form of a therapeutic community – in such a unit, the patients meet several times a day for group discussions, in which each person's behaviour and feelings are examined by the other group members.

2   Dialectical behaviour therapy (DBT):
  (a) Can be useful for parasuicidal patients with borderline personality disorder (BPD).
  (b) DBT encourages patients to take a non-judgemental approach to events and interactions and to do what is effective in situations, cf. to do what they may feel is 'right' in situations.
  (c) In the short term (first few months of treatment) – there is a dramatic improvement in self-harming behaviour.
  (d) In the longer term – results are less satisfactory; this suggests that DBT is more focused on reducing a single behavioural outburst of parasuicide, cf. altering the actual personality status of the patient.

IV **General measures:**
  1 The treatment plan aims to bring about limited changes in the patient's circumstances, so that he has less contact with situations that provoke his difficulties, and more opportunity to develop the assets in his personality.
  2 Admission to hospital should be avoided whenever possible, but may be necessary for short periods of crisis.

Prognosis

I   Personality disorders tend to become rather less disordered as the patient grows older.
II Patients with antisocial personality disorders over the age of 45 present fewer problems of aggressive behaviour than patients under the age of 45. However, their difficulties in personal relationships tend to persist.

CHAPTER 4
Anxiety disorders

Generalised anxiety disorder (GAD)

Definition

Various combinations of psychological and physical manifestations of anxiety, not attributable to real danger and occurring as a persisting state. Other neurotic features may be present (obsessional symptoms) but do not dominate the clinical picture. GAD is a long-term illness (minimum six months' symptoms) which is likely to require long-term treatment.

Epidemiology

I   Onset in the early twenties is not unusual. There is some evidence that phobias predict GAD in later life.
II Approximately twice as common in women.
III Lifetime prevalence: 4–6%.
IV Yearly prevalence: 2–3% (community samples).

Clinical features

I   Psychological symptoms and signs – fearful anticipation; irritability; a feeling of restlessness; sensitivity to noise; repetitive worrying thoughts; difficulty in concentration; subjective report of poor memory.
II Physical symptoms:
    1 **Respiratory symptoms** – difficulty in inhaling (cf. difficulty in expiration in asthma); feeling of constriction in the chest; overbreathing and its consequences – feeling of weakness; feeling of breathlessness; faintness; numbness; tinnitus; tingling in hands, feet and face; dizziness; headache; carpopedal spasms; precordial discomfort.

2   **Cardiovascular symptoms** – feeling of discomfort or pain over the heart; palpitations; throbbing in the neck; awareness of missed beats.

3   **Gastrointestinal symptoms** – excessive wind caused by aerophagy; borborygmi; difficulty in swallowing; dry mouth; epigastric discomfort; frequent or loose motions.

4   **Genito-urinary symptoms** – increased frequency and urgency of micturition; increased menstrual discomfort and amenorrhoea (in women); failure of erection; lack of libido.

5   **Neurological symptoms (related to central nervous system [CNS])** – tinnitus; dizziness; prickling sensations; blurring of vision.

6   **Musculo-skeletal symptoms** – aching and stiffness – especially in back and shoulders; trembling hands – impaired delicate movements; headache.

7   **Sleep disturbance** – difficulty getting off to sleep; after eventually falling asleep, patient wakes intermittently; often unpleasant dreams experienced; occasionally 'night terrors' experienced – in which patient wakes suddenly feeling intensely fearful.

Aetiology

I   **Genetic** – evidence for a genetic aetiology provided by:
1   **Family studies** – prevalence rate of the disorder in relatives of patients with anxiety disorders (generalised anxiety disorder and panic disorder) is 15% (cf. yearly prevalence of disorder in general population of 2–3%).
2   **Twin studies** (Slater and Shields) – 50% of monozygotic (MZ) twins concordant for anxiety disorders (generalised anxiety disorder/panic disorder) cf. only 2.5% concordance in dizygotic (DZ) twins.

II   **Biochemical and endocrine investigations:**
1   Increased secretions of adrenaline and noradrenaline in anxious patients.
2   Higher lactate levels after exercise in patients with anxiety disorders (generalised anxiety disorder and panic disorder), cf. normal subjects.

III **Psychoanalytic theory** – anxiety is experienced for the first time during the process of birth (primary anxiety). The child is overwhelmed by stimulation at the very moment of separation from its mother. This may explain why maternal separation can cause anxiety disorders.

IV   **Learning theory** – explains the tendency to develop excessive anxiety in terms of an inherited predisposition that is:
1   Reflected in undue lability of the autonomic nervous system.
2   Detected by measures of neuroticism.

Differential diagnosis

I   Exclude organic disorders in which anxiety symptoms occur – pre-senile and senile dementia; alcohol and drug abuse; thyrotoxicosis; phaeo-chromocytoma; hypoglycaemia.

II Exclude functional psychiatric illnesses in which anxiety symptoms occur:

1 Panic disorder – worry is about the possible occurrence or implications of panic attacks.

2 Social anxiety disorder – worry is about the negative evaluations by others.

3 Obsessive compulsive disorder – worry and anxiety is associated with intrusive thoughts, images or impulses that are distressing to the patient.

4 Hypochondriacal disorder – worry is about having a serious illness.

5 Depressive disorder –
  (a) Generalised anxiety occurs commonly.
  (b) It shares some associated symptoms – sleep disturbance/fatigue/restlessness/poor concentration.
  (c) GAD is not diagnosed if its features occur exclusively during a mood disorder (in DSM-IV).

6 Schizophrenia – anxiety symptoms may be a feature of the prodromal illness.

7 Anorexia nervosa – worry is about gaining weight.

Management

Goals of treatment – remission of symptoms and restoration of normal social functioning.

I   **Physical:**

1 **Benzodiazepines**
  (a) For decades – the most frequently prescribed medication for GAD.
  (b) Relatively few side-effects/safe/fast-acting.
  (c) Two-thirds of patients show moderate or marked improvement; effects are evident within one or two weeks of treatment.
  (d) More effective for somatic symptoms of anxiety, cf. psychic symptoms of anxiety – possibly due to their sedative and myorelaxant properties.
  (e) May increase irritability – therefore may be better for patients with mainly somatic complaints.

(f) Dose range for diazepam: 2 mg t.d.s. increased if necessary to 15–30 mg daily in divided doses.

(g) Indicated for short-term treatment of GAD; long-term treatment is associated with the risk of drug dependency – therefore benzodiazepines should not be used for more than four weeks.

2 **Buspirone**

(a) In recent years – popular alternative to benzodiazepines.

(b) Does not potentiate the effects of alcohol, cf. benzodiazepines, which do.

(c) Lacks sedative and myorelaxant properties of benzodiazepines.

(d) Improvement is slower over two to four weeks, cf. benzodiazepines.

(e) As effective as benzodiazepines for GAD.

(f) May reduce depression and agitation associated with GAD – therefore may be better for patients with mainly psychic complaints.

(g) Usual dose range 5 mg t.d.s. to 10 mg t.d.s.; maximum dose 15 mg t.d.s.

(h) Indicated for short-term treatment (up to several months) of GAD; long-term efficacy is untested.

(i) Physical dependence and abuse liability low, cf. benzodiazepines in which both psychic and physical dependence occur.

3 **Antidepressants**

(a) Tricyclic antidepressants (TCAs) and related antidepressants (imipramine and trazodone) – as effective as diazepam in reducing anxiety after two weeks of treatment.

(b) Serotonin and noradrenaline re-uptake inhibitors (SNRIs) (venlafaxine XL):

(i) As effective as buspirone.

(ii) Decline in anxiety evident in some cases by end of first week of treatment.

(iii) Dosage: 75 mg daily in UK; 75 mg to 225 mg daily in USA.

(iv) Approved for both the short-term and long-term treatment of moderate-to-severe GAD.

(v) Continued treatment appears to increase its benefits in terms of both response and remission.

(vi) Effective in the prevention of relapse of GAD.

(c) Selective serotonin re-uptake inhibitors (SSRIs) (paroxetine):

(i) Paroxetine is the first SSRI to have a licence for the treatment of GAD.

(ii) Dosage: 20 mg mane in UK; 20 mg to 50 mg mane in USA.

(iii) Approved for both the short-term and long-term treatment of GAD.

4   **Antipsychotics (chlorpromazine)** – have limited use as a short-term adjunctive treatment of severe anxiety.
5   **Psychosurgery** – reserved for cases of chronic, intractable, incapacitating anxiety, unresponsive to other measures (at least two years of treatment with other measures should be tried).
II   **Social** – social intervention aimed at current situational stresses.
III **Psychological:**
  1   **Behavioural therapy:**
    (a)   Relaxation training – this can take several forms:
      (i)   A procedure using a simple system of exercises intended to bring about progressive relaxation of individual groups of skeletal muscles and to regulate breathing.
      (ii) A procedure using a simple system of taped instruction intended to bring about relaxation – it is usual to link the resulting relaxed state with a pleasant, imagined scene so that relaxation can be induced in any situation merely by recalling the imagined scene.
    Such simple relaxation is effective in reducing mild-to-moderate anxiety, but not severe anxiety.
    (b)   Anxiety management training (AMT) – this procedure involves two stages:
      (i)   Verbal cues and mental imagery are used to arouse anxiety.
      (ii) The patient is trained to reduce this anxiety by relaxation, distraction and reassuring self-statements.
    AMT may be more effective in reducing anxiety than simple relaxation training, especially if the positive self-statements are individualised and address the patient's specific fear-evoking cognitions.
  2   **Cognitive therapy:**
    (a)   Technique:
      (i)   Beck suggests that a person who habitually adopts ways of thinking with anxious 'cognitive distortions' will be more likely to become anxious when faced with minor problems.
      (ii) In cognitive therapy, the patient attempts 'cognitive restructuring', i.e. he/she attempts to identify, evaluate and change his/her distorted thoughts and associated behaviours.
    (b)   Indication: cognitive therapy is indicated in the treatment of generalised anxiety disorder.
  3   **Newer cognitive and cognitive behavioural treatments:**
    (a)   In recent years – treatments have been developed that specifically target cognitive (e.g. worry) and behavioural (e.g. avoidance) features of GAD.
    (b)   About 12 sessions of treatment are required.

(c)   Either a group or individual format may be used.
(d)   These treatments are at least as effective as benzodiazepines.
(e)   Currently – the most successful treatments combine relaxation training with cognitive interventions, focused on making the worry process more controllable.
NB: *Combined pharmacotherapy and psychotherapy is common in clinical practice; however, there is little published data.*

Prognosis

I   Anxiety disorders (generalised anxiety disorder and panic disorder) of recent onset – most recover quickly.
II Anxiety disorders (generalised anxiety disorder and panic disorder) lasting more than six months – 80% are present three years later despite efforts at treatment.
III Poor prognosis is associated with – agitation; derealisation; syncopal episodes; suicidal ideas; hysterical features.
IV Patients who complain of physical symptoms are less easy to treat than those who recognise the emotional basis for their disorder.

Panic disorder (PD)

Definition

Various combinations of psychological and physical manifestations of anxiety, not attributable to real danger and occurring in attacks (panic attacks). Other features of anxiety disorders may be present (e.g. obsessional symptoms) but do not dominate the clinical picture.

Epidemiology

I   Average age of onset is early to mid-twenties. PD is bimodally distributed with an early presentation in the age range 15–24 years and a later presentation in the age range 45–54 years.
II Approximately twice as common in women.
III Lifetime prevalence: 1.5–2.5%.
IV Yearly prevalence: 1% (community samples).

Clinical features

The symptoms of panic attacks in order of their frequency:
I   Palpitations.
II   Pounding heart.
III   Tachycardia.
IV   Sweating.
V   Trembling or shaking.
VI   Shortness of breath or smothering.
VII   Feeling of choking.
VIII   Chest pain or discomfort.
IX   Nausea or abdominal distress.
X   Feeling dizzy, unsteady, light-headed or faint.
XI   Derealisation or depersonalisation.
XII   Fear of losing control or going mad.
XIII   Fear of dying.
XIV   Paraesthesias.
XV   Chills or hot flushes.

Aetiology

See aetiology of GAD.

Differential diagnosis

I   Exclude organic disorders:
   1   Cardiac conditions – arrhythmias; mitral valve prolapse (MVP).
   2   Respiratory conditions – chronic obstructive pulmonary disease (COPD).
   3   Neurological conditions – seizures.
   4   Endocrine disorders – hyperthyroidism; phaeochromocytoma.
   5   Substance abuse – alcohol; caffeine; amphetamines; cocaine.
II   Exclude functional psychiatric illnesses:
   1   Generalised anxiety disorder – patient has multiple, unrealistic and excessive worries about most aspects of life, not just panic attacks.
   2   Specific phobias – involve panic attacks, but they occur in the presence of a specific object (e.g. spiders, dogs) or in a specific situation (e.g. heights, thunderstorms, darkness).

3   Social anxiety disorder – patient has worries that are confined entirely to social situations, cf. the worries centring around the occurrence of panic attacks in PD.

4   Obsessive compulsive disorders – can involve panic attacks, but they occur in the specific context of obsessional concerns and are belittled in importance by typical obsessions and compulsive rituals.

5   Post-traumatic stress disorder – patient may have many panic-like symptoms, but their illness begins quite specifically after an extreme stress or life-threatening event.

6   Hypomania – can present with panic attacks.

Management

I   Physical:

1   SSRI

(a)   Paroxetine –

(i)   The first SSRI to have a licence for the treatment of PD (with or without agoraphobia).

(ii)   Dosage: 10 mg mane; this may be increased up to 50 mg daily in adults by weekly 10 mg increments if necessary.

(iii) Principal drawback – initial activation i.e. during the initial treatment of panic disorder, there is potential for a worsening of the panic symptoms; hence the starting dose of paroxetine of 10 mg mane in PD, cf. the starting dose of paroxetine of 20 mg mane in all its other indications.

(b)   Citalopram – dosage: 10 mg daily; this may be increased up to 60 mg daily in adults by weekly 10 mg increments if necessary; however, the usual recommended dose is 20–30 mg daily.

(c)   Escitalopram – starting dose 5 mg daily for one week; dosage: 10–20 mg daily.

2   **Benzodiazepines (alprazolam)**

(a)   Alprazolam is the most extensively studied benzodiazepine for PD.

(b)   The greatest difference with alprazolam is the rapid response, with some patients responding within the first few days of treatment.

(c)   Benzodiazepines remain the most frequently prescribed medication for PD world-wide.

(d)   Principal drawback – their abuse potential.

NB: Other benzodiazepines demonstrated to be effective in the treatment of PD include clonazepam, diazepam and lorazepam.

3 TCAs (imipramine and clomipramine)
   (a) Imipramine – may have a specific effect on autonomic reactivity in PD (where the starting dose is 25 mg).
   (b) Clomipramine – has been reported in low doses to have a specific action against panic symptoms (owing to it being a more selective re-uptake inhibitor of serotonin, cf. the other TCAs).
   (c) Principal drawbacks – initial activation/side-effects/dangerous in overdose.
4 **Monoamine oxidase inhibitors (MAOIs) (phenelzine and tranylcypromine)**
   (a) Some evidence for usefulness of MAOIs in PD – owing to anxiolytic properties.
   (b) Principal drawbacks – dietary restrictions/hypertensive crises.
5 **Reversible inhibitors of monoamine oxidase type A (RIMAs) (moclobemide)**
   (a) Has also been used in the treatment of PD.
   (b) Fewer concerns regarding its dietary restrictions, cf. conventional MAOIs.
II **Social** – social intervention aimed at current situational stresses.
III **Psychological:**
1 **Behavioural therapy:**
   (a) Relaxation training – *see* psychological management of GAD.
   NB: Relaxation training is useful in the management of PD, as long as it is combined with exposure tasks and the patient is taught how to apply it (applied relaxation).
   (b) Exposure treatments:
        (i)   Utilise *in vivo* exposure to phobic situations.
        (ii) Patients who enter a phobic situation experience habituation of their anxiety – whether they are exposed slowly (gradual exposure) or exposed suddenly and extensively (flooding).
        (iii) Principal drawbacks – many patients remain symptomatic; many studies report a patient drop-out of 10–25%.
2 **Cognitive therapy:**
   (a) Patients with PD interpret physical symptoms in a catastrophic way – these cognitive distortions need to be challenged and corrected.
   (b) Treatment involves an initial education component, followed by identification of these misinterpretations of panic symptoms.
   (c) Patients are then taught ways in which they can challenge and correct these misinterpretations.

(d) Most cognitive therapy is also combined with *in vivo* exposure to the physical symptoms that frighten them, e.g. a patient who is phobic of dizziness could be spun in a chair.

(e) Cognitive therapy when combined with *in vivo* exposure has been demonstrated to be more effective than applied relaxation.

(f) Cognitive therapy when combined with *in vivo* exposure has also been demonstrated in several studies to be more effective than medication – although this remains controversial.

Prognosis

See prognosis of GAD.

Phobic anxiety disorders

Definition

Anxiety states with an abnormally intense dread of certain objects or specific situations, which would not normally have that effect. The dread is accompanied by a strong wish to avoid the feared objects or situations.

Epidemiology

I   Specific phobias (include animal phobias):
   1   Onset in childhood for animal phobias; onset in early adult life for other specific phobias.
   2   More common among women.
II Agoraphobia:
   1   Onset usually between ages 15 and 35.
   2   More common among women.
III Social anxiety disorder (social phobia) (SAD):
   1   Onset usually between ages 17 and 30.
   2   Equally common in men and women.

Clinical features

I Specific phobias:
1 Some specific object or situation causes the person unreasonable anxiety, e.g. spiders, dogs, heights, thunderstorms, darkness.
2 There are three components:
   (a) Anxiety symptoms identical to those of any other anxiety state.
   (b) Anxious thoughts usually in anticipation of situations the person may have to encounter.
   (c) The habit of avoiding situations that provoke anxiety.
II Agoraphobia:
1 Strictly a fear of open spaces – but often used for a fear of:
   (a) Shops and supermarkets.
   (b) Buses and trains.
   (c) Crowds.
   (d) Any place that cannot be left suddenly without attracting attention, e.g. a seat in the middle of a row in the theatre.
2 The anxiety symptoms are identical to those of any other anxiety state. However, the associated anxious thoughts are characteristically centred on ideas of fainting or losing control.
3 As the condition progresses, the patient increasingly avoids the places or situations that provoke anxiety, so that only a few local shops can be reached.
4 In the most severe cases, the patient cannot leave the house at all – this condition is known as the housebound housewife syndrome.
5 Certain other non-phobic symptoms are common among agoraphobic patients – depersonalisation, depression, obsessions.
III SAD:
1 A fear of, and habit of avoiding, situations in which the individual may be observed by other people (e.g. restaurants, dinner parties, public transport). Also a fear that the individual may behave in a manner that will be humiliating or embarrassing (e.g. blushing, shaking).
2 The anxiety symptoms are identical to those of any other anxiety state.
3 The anxious thoughts are usually in anticipation of situations the person may have to encounter.
4 Certain other non-phobic symptoms occur among patients with SAD – depersonalisation, depression, obsessions (less frequent than in agoraphobic patients).

Aetiology

I   **Specific phobias:**
Psychoanalytic theory – the manifest fear is the symbolic representation of an unconscious conflict, i.e. the specific phobias represent some other source of anxiety that has been excluded from consciousness by repression and displacement.

II **Agoraphobia:**
   1   Psychoanalytic theory – when unconscious conflicts are not allowed direct expression because of repression, this may be transformed by displacement into phobias.
   2   Learning theory – agoraphobia develops as a series of conditioned fear responses with learned avoidance.

III **SAD** – the main reasons why a patient should develop a social phobia rather than some other kind could be:
   1   The circumstances in which the first episode of acute anxiety was experienced.
   2   General lack of self-confidence in social encounters.

Differential diagnosis

I   **Specific phobias** – seldom present difficulties of differential diagnosis.
II **Agoraphobia** – exclude: GAD; PD; SAD; depressive disorders; delusional disorders.
III **SAD** – exclude: social inadequacy; personality disorders; GAD; PD; depressive disorders; schizophrenia.

Management

I   **Physical**
   1   **Benzodiazepines** – provide some immediate relief of phobic symptoms in the short term.
   2   **TCAs** – effective due to their anxiolytic properties; more specifically, some clinicians consider imipramine to be the treatment of choice in agoraphobia.
   3   **MAOIs** – reduce agoraphobic symptoms, but there is a high relapse rate when drugs are stopped; moclobemide is also indicated in the treatment of phobic anxiety disorders (particularly SAD).

4 SSRIs
   (a) Paroxetine –
        (i)   The first SSRI to have a licence for the treatment of agora-
              phobia associated with PD (*see* physical management of PD).
        (ii) The first SSRI to have a licence for the treatment of SAD
              (dosage: 20 mg mane; if no improvement after at least two
              weeks, this may be increased up to 50 mg daily in adults by
              weekly 10 mg increments if necessary).
   (b) Citalopram – licensed for the treatment of agoraphobia asso-
        ciated with PD (*see* physical management of PD).
   (c) Escitalopram –
        (i)   Licensed for the treatment of agoraphobia associated with
              PD (*see* physical management of PD).
        (ii) Licensed for the treatment of SAD in 2004 (usual dosage
              10 mg daily; dose range 5–20 mg daily).

II Social – lasting improvement requires attention to the accompanying
    avoidance behaviour. In cases of recent onset, the patient should be
    encouraged to make determined efforts to go out more.

III Psychological:
   1 Systematic desensitisation (SD) in imagination:
      (a) Technique:
           (i)   Patients are required to imagine the anxiety-provoking
                 objects or situation vividly, starting with those that evoke
                 little fear and progressing through carefully planned stages
                 (a 'hierarchy') until the patient habituates, i.e. becomes
                 accustomed to the anxiety by frequent exposure, and the
                 avoidance response is extinguished.
           (ii) At each stage, anxiety is neutralised by relaxation training
                 (*see* relaxation training under the section 'Psychological
                 management of GAD', p. 21).
      (b) Indication: effective in the treatment of specific phobias of an
           object or situation not encountered readily (e.g. aeroplanes).
   2 Exposure *in vivo*:
      (a) Technique:
           (i)   Patients are exposed to the cues or triggers of anxiety-
                 provoking objects or situations, with a similar progression
                 up the 'hierarchy' as described in systematic desensitisation
                 in imagination, using real-life situations in a graded manner
                 of exposure.
           (ii) Habituation can be enhanced by simple anxiety manage-
                 ment techniques.

(b) Indications:
  (i) Effective in the treatment of specific phobias of an object or situation encountered readily.
  (ii) Effective in the treatment of agoraphobia, when it is combined with training patients to overcome avoidance behaviour in a planned way, the practice of which is carried out each day. This total package of treatment is known as programmed practice and is the treatment of choice in agoraphobia.

  NB: *In agoraphobia, the spouse can often be used as a co-therapist.*

3 **Group psychotherapy** – indicated in people with difficulties in social-isation (including SAD); group psychotherapy may offer them an opportunity to learn how to interact with other people.

Prognosis

I   **Specific phobias** – among adults, severe cases have usually persisted since childhood and continued for many years.

II   **Agoraphobia** – cases that have lasted for one year usually change little over the next five years.

III **SAD** – cases that have lasted for one year usually change little over the next five years; but many improve gradually over a longer period.

Obsessive compulsive disorder (OCD)

Definition

I   **Obsessions** – *see* Chapter 2.

II   **Compulsions** – the motor component of an obsessional thought.

Epidemiology

I   Onset is most commonly in early adult life.

II   Equally common among men and women.

III Prevalence rate of 0.05%.

Clinical features

I Obsessions – can occur in several forms:
   1 **Obsessional thoughts** – repeated and intrusive words or phrases, which are usually upsetting to the patient, e.g. violent, sexual and blasphemous themes.
   2 **Obsessional ruminations** – repeated worrying themes of a more complex kind, e.g. about the world ending.
   3 **Obsessional doubts** – repeated themes expressing uncertainty about previous actions, e.g. whether or not the person turned off a gas tap that might cause a fire.
   4 **Obsessional impulses** – repeated urges to carry out actions that are usually dangerous, aggressive or socially embarrassing, e.g. to shout obscenities in church.
   5 **Obsessional phobias** – obsessional thoughts with a fearful content, e.g. 'I must have AIDS'; or obsessional impulses that lead to anxiety and avoidance, e.g. the impulse to stab someone with a knife and the consequent avoidance of knives.
II Compulsions:
   1 Also known as *compulsive rituals*.
   2 A compulsion is usually associated with an obsession as if it has the function of reducing the distress caused by the obsession, e.g. obsessional thoughts that the hands are contaminated with faecal matter are often followed by a handwashing compulsion.
III **Obsessional slowness** – usually the result of obsessional doubts or compulsive rituals.

Aetiology

I **Genetic** – some evidence for a genetic aetiology is provided by:
   1 **Family studies** – disorder occurs in 5–7% of the parents of patients with obsessive compulsive disorder, cf. a prevalence rate of 0.05% in the general population.
   2 **Twin studies** – concordance of the disorder in MZ twins is 50–80%; cf. concordance in DZ twins of 25%.
II **Organic factors** – some evidence for organic brain disease is provided by the frequency of obsessional symptoms observed in patients after the epidemic of encephalitis lethargica.
III **Premorbid personality** – 70% of patients with obsessive compulsive disorders have premorbid anankastic personality traits – cleanliness, orderliness, rigid checking.

IV Psychoanalytic theory (Freud):
1   Obsessional symptoms result from repressed impulses of an aggressive or sexual nature.
2   Obsessional symptoms occur as a result of regression to the anal stage of psychosexual development.
V   **Learning theory** – suggests that obsessional thoughts occurring with rituals are the equivalent of avoidance responses.

Differential diagnosis

Exclude other disorders in which obsessional symptoms occur: GAD; PD; phobic anxiety disorders; depressive disorders; schizophrenia; organic disorders.

Management

I   Physical:
1   **Benzodiazepines** – provide some short-term symptomatic relief of obsessive compulsive symptoms (should not be prescribed for more than 2–4 weeks' duration).
2   **TCAs** – appropriate when anxiolytic treatment has to be prolonged beyond the few (2–4) weeks for which benzodiazepines are prescribed; more specifically, it has been reported that clomipramine has a specific action against obsessional symptoms (owing to its being a more selective re-uptake inhibitor of serotonin, cf. the other TCAs).
3   **SSRIs** – indicated in the treatment of obsessive compulsive disorders (OCD); there are four SSRIs currently with a licence in the UK to treat OCD:
(a)   Fluvoxamine – dose range: 50 mg o.d. to 150 mg b.d.
(b)   Fluoxetine – dose range: 20 mg mane to 80 mg mane; increasing the dosage within this range increasingly targets obsessional symptoms.
(c)   Paroxetine – dosage: 20 mg mane; this may be increased up to 60 mg daily in adults by weekly 10 mg increments if necessary; it may be the SSRI of choice to treat OCD, owing to its established anxiolytic profile and anti-obsessional effect.
(d)   Sertraline – dose range: 50 mg mane to 200 mg mane.
4   **Buspirone** – may be useful in the treatment of obsessive compulsive disorder as an augmenting agent to SSRIs.

5   **Antipsychotics** – small doses of chlorpromazine of value when anxiolytic treatment is needed for more than the 2–4 weeks' duration for which benzodiazepines are prescribed.

6   **Psychosurgery** – reserved for cases of chronic, intractable, incapacitating illness, unresponsive to other measures (at least two years of treatment with other measures should be tried).

II   **Social** – obsessional patients often involve other family members in their rituals. In planning treatment it is essential to interview relatives and encourage them to adopt a firm but sympathetic attitude to the patient.

III   **Psychological:**

1   **Supportive psychotherapy** – the supportive relationship any member of the multidisciplinary team has with a patient; the primary aim is to maintain their functioning capacity, maintain their defences and strengths and help promote their adaptation to everyday living; it can also benefit patients by providing continuing hope.

2   **Flooding and response prevention:**

(a)   Technique:

(i)   The technique involves exposing the patient to a contaminating object such as a toilet seat or a soiled towel, i.e. exposing the patient to those situations previously evoking compulsive rituals (flooding).

(ii)   The patient is subsequently prevented from carrying out the usual compulsive cleansing rituals until the urge to do so has passed (response prevention).

(b)   Indications:

(i)   The combination of flooding and response prevention is the behavioural treatment of choice in the treatment of obsessional thoughts occurring with compulsive rituals – with persistence, the compulsive rituals and the distress subsequently diminish.

(ii)   The obsessional thoughts accompanying the rituals usually improve as well with this treatment.

3   **Thought stopping:**

(a)   Technique:

(i)   The patient is asked to ruminate and, upon doing so, the therapist immediately shouts 'stop' to teach the patient to interrupt the intrusive, obsessional thoughts.

(ii)   After considerable practice the patient learns to internalise the 'stop' order so that the thought-stopping technique can be used outside the therapy situation.

(iii)   Alternatively, the patient can arrest the obsessional thoughts by arranging a sudden intrusion, such as snapping an elastic band on the wrist.

(b) Indication: thought stopping is indicated in the treatment of obsessional ruminative thoughts occurring without compulsive rituals.

Prognosis

I   Two-thirds of cases improve by the end of one year.
II   Cases lasting more than one year usually run a fluctuating course, with periods of partial or complete remission lasting a few months to several years.
III   Poor prognosis is associated with:
    1   Anankastic personality traits.
    2   Continuing stressful events in patient's life.
    3   Severe symptoms.

Acute stress reaction or disorder

Definition

I   ICD-10: acute stress reaction – brief response (lasting from several hours to about three days) to severely stressful events.
II   DSM-IV: acute stress disorder – a more prolonged response (lasting from at least two days to at most four weeks) to severely stressful events.

Epidemiology

Rate of acute stress disorder reported:
I   Among survivors of motor vehicle accidents – 13%.
II   Among victims of violent crime – 19%.
III   Among witnesses of a mass shooting – 33%.

Clinical features

I   Core symptoms of an acute stress reaction or disorder:
    1   Anxiety – the response to threatening experiences.
    2   Depression – the response to loss.
II   Other symptoms of an acute stress reaction or disorder include:
    1   A sense of numbing or detatchment.

2 A sense of 'being in a daze'.
3 Insomnia.
4 Poor concentration.
5 Restlessness.
6 Anger or histrionic behaviour.
7 Physical symptoms of autonomic arousal – especially sweating, tremor and palpitations.

III Coping strategies and defence mechanisms are also part of an acute stress reaction or disorder:

1 Avoidance is the most frequent coping strategy –
   (a) The person avoids talking or thinking about the severely stressful events.
   (b) The person avoids reminders of the severely stressful events.
   NB: Coping strategies may be maladaptive, e.g. excessive use of alcohol or drugs to reduce distress.

2 Denial is the most frequent defence mechanism –
   (a) Experienced as a belief that the severely stressful events have not really happened.
   (b) Experienced as an inability to remember the severely stressful events.
   NB: Defence mechanisms may be of the less adaptive types, e.g. regression, displacement or projection.

Aetiology

I Various kinds of severely stressful events can provoke an acute stress reaction or disorder:

1 Involvement in a significant but brief event, e.g. a motor vehicle accident.
2 An event that involves actual or threatened injury, e.g. a physical assault.
3 The sudden discovery of serious illness.

II Some of these severely stressful events may involve life changes to which further adjustment is required, e.g. the serious physical injury of a close friend or relative involved in the same motor vehicle accident.

Diagnostic conventions

I ICD-10: Acute stress reaction is a response to severely stressful events that starts within an hour of exposure and begins to diminish within no more than eight hours if the stressor is transient, or within no more than forty-eight hours if the stressor continues.

II   DSM-IV:

1   Acute stress disorder is a response to severely stressful events that starts while experiencing or after experiencing the events, and lasts at least two days to at most four weeks.

2   The DSM-IV definition refers to cases of more clinical importance and it is widely used, cf. the ICD-10 definition.

3   In DSM-IV the diagnosis of acute stress disorder requires fear, helplessness, or horror, together with three of the following five 'dissociative' symptoms:

(a)   A sense of numbing or detachment.

(b)   A sense of 'being in a daze' (reduced awareness of the surroundings).

(c)   Depersonalisation.

(d)   Derealisation.

(e)   Dissociative amnesia.

4   DSM-IV requires there must be avoidance of stimuli that arouse recollections of the severely stressful events, and significant distress or impaired social functioning.

III   The diagnosis of acute stress reaction or disorder can only be made if the person was free from psychiatric disorder at the time of impact of the severely stressful events; otherwise the response is classified as an exacerbation of pre-existing psychiatric disorder.

Management

The management of an acute stress reaction or disorder has three components:

I   Reducing the emotional response:

1   This can often be achieved if the affected person talks informally to sympathetic relatives or friends, or to members of the professional staff dealing with the consequences of the severely stressful events, e.g. physical injury resulting from a motor vehicle accident.

2   More formal counselling may be required:

(a)   If there is no confidant.

(b)   If the severely stressful events cannot easily be discussed with sympathetic relatives or friends e.g. some cases of rape.

(c)   If the response to the acute stress reaction or disorder is prolonged or severe.

   3 When anxiety is severe: an anxiolytic drug may be prescribed for one or two days.

   4 When sleep is severely disrupted: a hypnotic drug may be prescribed for one or two nights.

   5 There is evidence that cognitive behavioural techniques are more effective, cf. supportive counselling.

II Encouraging recall (debriefing):

   1 Discussion of the severely stressful events helps to prevent the persistence of the coping strategy of avoidance and/or the defence mechanism of denial, which may prolong or intensify the problem.

   2 Gradual repeated questioning may be needed to help the person remember the severely stressful events and express the associated feelings.

III Learning effective coping skills – if there has been an acute crisis for which coping strategies have been maladaptive (e.g. excessive use of alcohol or drugs to reduce distress), there may be an opportunity for the person to learn how to adopt effective coping strategies in future with crisis intervention counselling.

Prognosis

I   78% of people who meet the DSM-IV criteria for acute stress disorder go on to develop PTSD (*see* next section).

II 60% of people who fail to meet the DSM-IV criteria for acute stress disorder go on to develop PTSD.

Post-traumatic stress disorder (PTSD)

Definition

PTSD begins quite specifically after an extreme stress or life-threatening event, where the patient feels threatened with death or serious injury. The patient may experience many panic-like symptoms. PTSD does not affect everyone who is exposed to this event; it only affects those who are thought to be more vulnerable individuals.

Epidemiology

Lifetime prevalence – 11% in women
5% in men.

Clinical features

I   Direct exposure to an extreme stress or life-threatening event – leading to the development of characteristic anxiety symptoms.
II Psychological impairment – in most patients the onset of PTSD occurs shortly after exposure to the traumatic event; however, PTSD can present up to six months after the traumatic event (ICD-10 criterion).
III Recurrent reliving of the traumatic event – recurrent nightmares/flashbacks.
IV Phobic avoidance of stimuli associated with the traumatic event – a restricted range of interest and affect.
V   Symptoms of hyperarousal – hypervigilance/characteristic startle response.

Aetiology

I   Any traumatic event can act as a trigger – the more life-threatening, longer lasting and unavoidable the traumatic event, the greater the likelihood of developing PTSD.
II Well-recognised situations for developing PTSD include:
   1   Exposure to high combat in Vietnam and other wars.
   2   Exposure to natural disasters, e.g. Hillsborough deaths.
   3   Rape.
   4   Physical assault.
   5   Road traffic accidents (RTAs).
III Predisposing factors include:
   1   PPH.
   2   Previous exposure to traumatic events.
IV Biochemical and endocrine abnormalities in patients with PTSD include:
   1   Central noradrenergic dysfunction – hyperresponsivity of noradrenergic neurones.
   2   Increased glucocorticoid receptor sensitivity.
   3   Chronic low hydrocortisone levels.

Comorbidity

Increased risk of:
I   Personality disorders.
II   PD.
III   Specific phobias.
IV   Agoraphobia.
V   SAD.
VI   OCD.
VII   Depressive disorder.
VIII   Substance abuse.

Management

I   Physical:
   1   SSRIs (paroxetine/sertraline) –
     (a)   Paroxetine –
       (i)   The first SSRI to have a licence for the treatment of PTSD.
       (ii) Dosage: 20 mg mane; this may be increased up to 50 mg daily in adults by gradual 10 mg increments if necessary.
     (b)   Sertraline –
       (i)   Licensed for the treatment of post-traumatic stress disorder in women only.
       (ii) Starting dose 25 mg mane for one week; dose range: 50 mg mane to 200 mg mane.
   2   TCAs (amitriptyline/imipramine) – evidence for some efficacy.
   3   MAOIs (phenelzine) – evidence of efficacy but poor side-effect tolerability.
   4   Benzodiazepines – not generally used due to their abuse potential and the chronic nature of PTSD.
II   Psychological:
   1   Psychoeducation – an explanation to the patient about the stress, the nature of PTSD and its treatment options.
   2   Supportive psychotherapy.
   3   Group therapy.
   4   Early intervention and prevention with 'debriefing' – to avert the development of chronic PTSD.
   5   Behavioural treatments – exposure treatments, i.e. graded exposure to imagery of the traumatic event.
   6   Cognitive therapy.

Prognosis

Poor prognostic features:
I   Comorbidity.
II   Longer lasting symptoms of greater severity.
III   PPH.
IV   FPH.
V   Poor social support.
VI   Poor premorbid function.

Adjustment disorder

Definition

The psychological reactions involved in adapting to new circumstances, e.g.
divorce.

Epidemiology

I   Prevalence rate in hospital attenders in USA – estimated at 5%.
II   It is possible that a different prevalence rate would apply to the UK – where a
      greater proportion of adjustment disorders are treated in primary care.

Clinical features

I   Psychological symptoms:
      1   Anxiety.
      2   Irritability.
      3   Depression.
      4   Worry.
      5   Poor concentration.
II   Physical symptoms of autonomic arousal:
      1   Tremor.
      2   Palpitations.
III   Other clinical features may include:
      1   Excessive use of alcohol or drugs.
      2   Episodes of deliberate self-harm.
      3   Outbursts of dramatic or aggressive behaviour.

IV ICD-10 indicates that it usually starts within one month of the change of circumstances, cf. DSM-IV which indicates that it starts within three months of the change of circumstances.

V The onset is more gradual, cf. the onset of an acute stress reaction or disorder.

VI The course is more prolonged, cf. the course of an acute stress reaction or disorder.

VII Social functioning is usually impaired.

VIII The diagnosis of adjustment disorder is not made when the diagnostic criteria for another psychiatric disorder are met.

IX It is essential that the psychological reactions are understandably related to, and in proportion to, the change of circumstances, taking into account the patient's previous experiences and personality.

Aetiology

I Change of circumstances – the necessary cause of an adjustment disorder.

II Individual vulnerability – an important cause of an adjustment disorder since not all people exposed to the same change of circumstances develop an adjustment disorder; this may relate in part to previous life experiences.

Management

The management of an adjustment disorder has three components:

I Help resolve the change of circumstances if possible.

II Help the natural processes of adjustment by –
   1 Helping to prevent the persistence of the coping strategy of avoidance and/or the defence mechanism of denial, which may prolong or intensify the problem.
   2 Discouraging maladaptive coping strategies, e.g. excessive use of alcohol or drugs to reduce distress.
   3 Encouraging the patient to use problem-solving counselling to:
      (a) Seek solutions to the change of circumstances.
      (b) Consider the advantages and disadvantages of various courses of action, the patient then being helped to select and implement a course of action to problem-solve.

III Help relieve anxiety by encouraging the patient to talk about the change of circumstances and express the associated feelings.

NB: When anxiety is severe, an anxiolytic drug may be prescribed for one or two days; when sleep is severely disrupted, a hypnotic drug may be prescribed for one or two nights.

Prognosis

I   Most adjustment disorders last for several months.
II A few adjustment disorders persist for years.
III Adults with adjustment disorder have a good prognosis.
IV Some adolescents with adjustment disorder develop psychiatric disorder in adult life.

CHAPTER 5

Dissociative (conversion) disorders

Definition

I **Hysterical dissociation** – an apparent dissociation between different mental activities.
II **Hysterical conversion** – the term stems from Freud's theory that mental energy can be converted into certain physical symptoms.

Epidemiology

I Onset usually before the age of 35.
II Probably more common among women.
III More common in lower social classes.

Clinical features

I **Hysterical dissociation** – the major dissociative reactions are:
   1 Psychogenic amnesia.
   2 Psychogenic fugue (wandering).
   3 Somnambulism (sleepwalking).
   4 Multiple personality – sudden alternations between two patterns of behaviour, each of which is forgotten by the patient when the other is present.
II **Hysterical conversion** – 'classic' conversion symptoms are:
   1 Paralysis.
   2 Fits.
   3 Blindness.
   4 Deafness.

5   Aphonia.
6   Anaesthesia.
7   Abdominal pain.
8   Disorders of gait.
III **Primary gain** – anxiety arising from a psychological conflict is excluded from the patient's conscious mind.
IV **Secondary gain** – the symptoms of dissociative (conversion) disorders usually confer some advantage on the patient, e.g. the attention of others.
V **'Belle indifference'** – less than the expected amount of distress often shown by patients with hysterical symptoms.
VI **There are no demonstrable organic findings.**

Aetiology

I   **Genetic** – genetic aetiology unlikely since:
   1   **Family studies** – incidence among first-degree relatives of about 5% is higher than in the general population. However, this level most likely reflects family learning.
   2   **Twin Studies** (Slater) – in a sample of 12 MZ twins and 12 DZ twins, none were concordant for dissociative (conversion) disorders.
II **Premorbid personality** – 12–21% of patients with dissociative (conversion) disorders have premorbid histrionic personality traits (*see* Chapter 3)
III **Psychoanalytic theory (Freud):**
   1   Patients suffer from the effects of emotionally charged ideas lodged in the unconscious at some time in the past.
   2   Symptoms are explained as the combined effects of repression and the 'conversion' of psychic energy into physical channels.

Differential diagnosis

I   Exclude organic brain disease – for example:
   1   Dementia.
   2   Cerebral tumour.
   3   General paralysis of the insane (GPI).
   4   Multiple sclerosis.
   5   Complex, partial seizures (temporal lobe epilepsy).
II Exclude histrionic personality disorder.
III Exclude malingering – particularly among prisoners and military servicemen.

Management

I   **Physical** – abreaction
   1   Clasically, abreaction was brought about by an intravenous injection of small amounts of amylobarbitone sodium. Now, such abreaction can be initiated more safely by a slow intravenous injection of 10 mg of diazepam.
   2   In the resulting state, the patient is encouraged to relive the stressful events that provoked the dissociative (conversion) disorder, and to express the accompanying emotions.
II **Social:**
   1   **For acute cases lasting up to a few weeks** – treatment by reassurance and suggestion is usually appropriate, together with immediate efforts to resolve any stressful circumstances that provoked the reaction.
   2   **General approach** – to focus on the elimination of factors that are reinforcing the symptoms, and on the encouragement of normal behaviour.
III **Psychological** – psychotherapy:
   1   Patients usually respond well to exploratory psychotherapy concerned with their past life.
   2   They often produce striking memories of childhood sexual behaviour and other problems apparently relevant to dynamic psychotherapy.
   3   However, such ideas should not be explored at length since this may lead to over-dependence.

Prognosis

I   Cases of recent onset – recover quickly.
II Cases that last longer than one year are likely to persist for many years more.

CHAPTER 6

Hypochondriacal disorders

Definition

A disorder in which the conspicuous features are the patient's excessive concern with his health in general, in the integrity and functioning of some part of his body or, less frequently, his mind.

Epidemiology

More common among:
I Elderly.
II Men.
III Lower social classes.
IV Those closely associated with disease.

Clinical features

I Pain – common sites are:
    1 Right iliac fossa.
    2 Lower lumbar region.
    3 Head.
II Worries about bladder function.
III Complaints about appearance – especially the shape of the breasts, nose or ears.
IV Complaints about sweating or body odour.
V Cardiovascular symptoms:
    1 Dyspnoea.
    2 Left-sided chest pain.
    3 Palpitations.
    4 Worries about blood pressure.

VI Gastrointestinal symptoms:
1   Acid regurgitation.
2   Biliousness.
3   Nausea.
4   Bad taste in mouth.
5   Abdominal pain.
6   Flatulence.
7   Dysphagia.

Aetiology

Psychoanalytic theory:
I   An expression of anal eroticism.
II   A defence against psychosis.

Differential diagnosis

Exclude: personality disorders; GAD; PD; depressive disorders; schizophrenia; organic disorders – dementia.

Management

I   **Physical** – some advocate a trial of tricyclic antidepressants in all patients (especially if the patient is depressed).
II   **Social** – search for meaning of symptoms in social/family setting, where appropriate. Exercise caution where symptoms serve powerful defensive purposes.
III **Psychological** – supportive measures are the mainstay of treatment. Patients should be educated over the role of psychological factors in the symptoms. In addition, cognitive therapy is indicated in the treatment of hypochondriacal disorder.

Prognosis

I   More chronic and established cases – poor prognosis.
II   Cases associated with anxiety disorders or depressive disorders – better prognosis.

CHAPTER 7

Delusional disorders

Classification

I **Persistent delusional disorder** – A paranoid condition that is not associated with a primary organic, schizophrenic or affective disorder, in which delusions, especially of being influenced, persecuted or treated in some special way, are the main symptoms. The delusions are of a fairly fixed, elaborate and systematised kind.

II **Paranoia** – A permanent and unshakeable delusional system, developing insidiously in a person in middle or late life. The delusional system is encapsulated, hallucinations are absent and personality is intact. The patient can often go on working, and his social life may sometimes be maintained fairly well.

III **Paraphrenia** – The late onset of systematised delusion, with prominent hallucinations, and preservation of personality and intellect.

IV **Induced psychosis (folie à deux)** – A paranoid delusional system which appears to have developed in a person as a result of a close relationship with another person who already has an established and similar delusional system. The delusions are nearly always persecutory.

V **Special paranoid conditions:**
   1 **Othello syndrome:**
   (a) **Essential feature** – a delusional belief that the marital partner is being unfaithful.
   (b) **This may be accompanied by other delusions** – that the spouse is trying to poison the patient, plotting against him, infecting him with venereal disease, or taking away his sexual capacities.
   (c) **Behaviour** – intensive seeking for evidence of partner's infidelity, e.g. by examining sexual organs, underwear or bed-linen for signs of sexual secretions. The patient has the desire to extract a confession from the spouse. This may lead to severe aggression and murder.
   (d) **Mood** – mixture of anger, apprehension, irritability and misery.
   (e) **Epidemiology** – more common among men.
   (f) **Prognosis** – often poor.

2 De Clerambault's syndrome:
   (a) Essential feature – a delusional belief that another person (the object), often of unattainably higher social status, loves the patient (the subject) intensely.
   (b) The subject is usually a single woman.
   (c) The subject believes she has been specially chosen by the object, and that it was not she who made the initial advances.
   (d) The subject is convinced that the object cannot be happy or a complete person without her.
   (e) The subject believes that the object is unable to reveal his love to her.
   (f) The subject may be importunate and disrupt the object's life.
   (g) After rejection by the object, the subject's feelings may turn to hatred.
3 **Capgras' syndrome** – Essential feature – illusion de Sosies: a delusion in which a patient sees a familiar person and believes him to have been replaced by an impostor, who is an exact double of the original person.
4 **Fregoli's syndrome** – Essential feature – Fregoli's illusion: a delusion in which a patient recognises a number of people as having different appearances, but believes that they are all a single persecutor in disguise.
5 **Monosymptomatic hypochondriacal psychosis (MHP)** – Essential feature – hypochondriacal delusions: a delusion in which a patient is convinced of the physical cause of his complaint; he subsequently gathers 'evidence' for it.

Aetiology

I   **Paranoia:**
   1 Cases are rarely encountered.
   2 Psychoanalytic theory – associated with the ego-defence mechanisms projection and splitting.
II **Paraphrenia** – condition best regarded as paranoid schizophrenia of late onset and good prognosis.
III **Induced psychosis** – psychoanalytic theory – over-identification with psychotic person in a submissive over-dependent personality.
IV **Othello syndrome:**
   1 Usually associated with personality disorders or neuroses. Also associated with: depressive disorders; schizophrenia; organic disorders – e.g. alcoholism, drug abuse.
   2 Psychoanalytic theory:
      (a) Projection of own desires for infidelity.

      (b)   Projection of repressed homosexuality.
      (c)   The result of other feelings of inadequacy.
V   De Clerambault's syndrome:
    1   Usually associated with paranoid schizophrenia. Also associated with: affective disorders; organic disorders.
    2   Psychoanalytic theory – If 'pure' form (i.e. not associated with any other disorder): projection of denied, narcissistic self-love.
VI   Capgras' syndrome:
    1   Usually associated with affective disorders or schizophrenia. Rarely associated with organic disorders.
    2   Psychoanalytic theory – ambivalent attitude to the person implicated.
VII Fregoli's syndrome – Usually associated with schizophrenia.
VIII MHP:
    1   Often depressed or paranoid.
    2   Sometimes organic brain disorder.
    3   Occasionally an isolated phenomenon.

Management

I   Persistent delusional disorder:
    1   Physical:
      (a)   Symptoms are sometimes relieved by antipsychotic medication, e.g. chlorpromazine, haloperidol, trifluoperazine.
      (b)   Choice of drug and dosage depend on:
          (i)   Age of patient.
          (ii)   Physical condition of patient.
          (iii) Degree of agitation.
          (iv) Response to previous medication.
      (c)   Commonest cause of relapse – non-compliance with medication because patients suspect medication will harm them. It may then be necessary to prescribe a long-acting (depot) preparation, e.g. fluphenazine decanoate.
    2   Social – The psychiatrist should strive to maintain a good relationship with the patient. He or she should show compassionate interest in the patient's beliefs, but without condemning them or colluding in them.
    3   Psychological – Psychological support, encouragement and assurance.
II   Induced psychosis:
    1   Physical – Treat the psychotic member, if identifiable.

   2 **Social** – It is usually necessary to advise separation of the affected people. This sometimes leads to the disappearance of the delusional state, improvement being more likely in the recipient than the inducer.

   3 **Psychological** – Supportive psychotherapy and family therapy are often indicated.

III **Othello syndrome:**

   1 **Physical:**

   (a) Treatment of any underlying disorder.

   (b) In cases where underlying diagnosis is uncertain – phenothiazines (e.g. chlorpromazine) may be beneficial.

   2 **Social** – Geographical separation from partner often advisable.

   3 **Psychological:**

   (a) Psychotherapy:

   (i) Given to patients with personality disorders or anxiety disorders.

   (ii) Aims to reduce tensions by allowing the patient and spouse to ventilate feelings.

   (b) Behaviour therapy – encouraging the partner to produce behaviour that reduces jealousy, e.g. refusal to argue or counter-aggression.

IV **De Clerambault's syndrome:**

   1 Treatment of any underlying disorder.

   2 If 'pure' form – very resistant to physical treatment and psychotherapy

V **Capgras' syndrome** – Treatment of any underlying disorder.

VI **Fregoli's syndrome** – Treatment of any underlying disorder.

VII **MHP** – it is claimed that pimozide has success in specifically targeting monosymptomatic hypochondriacal delusions (dose range: 4–16 mg daily).

   1 Special caution is needed over rate of rise in daily doses.

   2 Following reports of sudden unexplained death, CSM recommends:

   (a) An ECG prior to commencing treatment in all patients.

   (b) An annual ECG in all patients on pimozide.

   (c) A review of the need for pimozide if arrhythmias develop.

CHAPTER 8

Affective disorders

Definition

Disorders characterised by mood disturbance (inappropriate depression or elation). Usually accompanied by abnormalities in thinking and perception arising out of the mood disturbance.

Classification

I   **Bipolar affective disorders** – Recurring attacks of both mania and depression. (At least one manic/hypomanic episode required to make this diagnosis.)
II **Unipolar affective disorders** (unipolar depression) – Recurring attacks of depression only.
III **Mixed affective states** – Cases where manic and depressive symptoms occur simultaneously.

Epidemiology

I   **Age** – depressive disorders:
    1 Women – highest prevalence rate between 35 and 45 years.
    2 Men – prevalence rate increases with age.
II **Sex:**
    1 Bipolar affective disorders – equally common among men and women.
    2 All depressive disorders – twice as common in women.
III **Social class** – More common in social classes I, II and V.
IV **Marital status** – More common among the divorced or separated.
V   **Prevalence rate** – 5% of the general population.

Clinical features

A   Depressive disorders

I   Biological features of depression:
  1 Sleep disturbance:
     (a)   Characteristically early morning wakening (middle insomnia) –
            occurs 2–3 hours before the patient's usual time. He does not
            fall asleep again, but lies awake feeling unrefreshed with de-
            pressive thinking.
     (b)   Also onset insomnia (initial insomnia) – delay in falling asleep.
     (c)   Some depressed patients sleep excessively (cf. waking early) –
            but still feel unrefreshed on waking.
  2 Change in appetite:
     (a)   Characteristically loss of appetite.
     (b)   Less commonly increased appetite.
  3 Change in weight:
     (a)   Characteristically loss of weight.
     (b)   Less commonly increased weight.
  4 Change in psychomotor activity:
     (a)   Characteristically psychomotor retardation (slowed up).
     (b)   Sometimes agitation.
  5 Diurnal variation in mood:
     (a)   Characteristically worse in the morning.
     (b)   Sometimes worse in the evening.
  6 Loss of interest in work and pleasure activities.
  7 Loss of energy and fatigue.
  8 Loss of libido.
  9 Change in bowel habit – constipation.
  10 Change in menstrual cycle – amenorrhoea.
II   Appearance:
  1   Neglected dress and grooming.
  2   Facial features:
     (a)   Turning downwards of corners of mouth.
     (b)   Vertical furrowing of centre of brow.
  3   Reduced rate of blinking.
  4   Reduced gestural movements.
  5   Shoulders bent, head inclined forwards, direction of gaze down-
        wards.
  NB: *Some patients maintain a smiling exterior while depressed.*

III   **Speech:**
    1   Poverty of speech.
    2   Hesitancy – long delay before questions are answered.

IV   **Mood:**
    1   One of misery.
    2   Qualitatively different from normal unhappiness.
    3   'Autonomous' – i.e. loss of reactivity to circumstances.
    4   Anxiety and irritability also occur.

V   **Thought:**
    1   Morbid thoughts:
      (a)   Concerned with the past – often take form of unreasonable guilt and self-blame about minor matters, e.g. feeling guilty about past trivial acts of dishonesty.
      (b)   Concerned with the present:
        (i)   The patient sees the unhappy side of every event.
        (ii)   He thinks he is failing in everything he does and that other people see him as a failure.
        (iii)   He no longer feels confident, and discounts any success as a chance happening for which he can take no credit.
      (c)   Concerned with the future:
        (i)   Ideas of hopelessness – the patient expects the worst.
        (ii)   Often accompanied by the thought that life is no longer worth living for and that death would come as a welcome release.
        (iii)   May progress to thoughts of, and plans for, suicide.
    2   Poverty of thought.

VI   **Psychotic features of depression:**
    1   Delusions:
      (a)   Delusions concerned with themes of worthlessness, guilt, ill-health, poverty, e.g. a patient with hypochondriacal delusions (i.e. delusions of ill-health) may be convinced that he has cancer.
      (b)   Persecutory delusions, e.g. the patient may believe that other people are about to take revenge on him. Typically the patient accepts the supposed persecution as something he has brought upon himself.
    2   Hallucinations:
      (a)   Usually second person auditory hallucinations – voices addressing repetitive words and phrases to the patient. The voices confirm the patient's ideas of worthlessness, e.g. 'you are an evil man; you should die', or make derisive comments, or urge the patient to take his own life.

    (b) A few patients experience visual hallucinations, sometimes in the form of scenes of death and destruction.

VII **Cognition:**
1 Impaired attention and concentration.
2 Poor memory.

VIII **Physical symptoms:**
1 Aching discomfort anywhere in the body.
2 Increased complaints about any pre-existing physical disorder.

IX **Other psychiatric symptoms:**
1 Phobic symptoms.
2 Obsessional symptoms.
3 Dissociative (conversion) symptoms.
4 Hypochondriacal preoccupations.
5 Depersonalisation.

B   Mania (hypomania)

I **Biological features of mania:**
1 Sleep disturbance – often reduced, but no fatigue. Patient wakes early feeling lively and energetic. Often, he gets up and busies himself noisily to the surprise of other people.
2 Change in appetite – increased appetite. Food may be eaten greedily with little attention to conventional manners.
3 Change in weight – weight loss due to overactivity.
4 Change in psychomotor activity – psychomotor acceleration (speeded up).
5 Diurnal variation in mood – though not with the regular rhythm characteristic of depressive disorders.
6 Increased drive in work and pleasure activities.
7 Increased energy without fatigue.
8 Increased libido – behaviour may be uninhibited. Women sometimes neglect precautions against pregnancy.

II **Appearance and behaviour:**
1 Clothing – bright colours and ill-assorted choice of garments.
2 Untidy and dishevelled appearance.
3 Overactivity – if persistent may lead to physical exhaustion.
4 Excessive activity in risk-taking pursuits; indiscretion socially.

III **Speech** – pressure of speech

IV **Mood:**
1 One of euphoria with infectious gaiety.
2 May be interrupted by brief episodes of depression.
3 Anger and irritability also occur.

V   Thought:
  1 Expansive ideas – patient believes that his ideas are original, his opinions important, and his work of outstanding quality.
  2 Pressure of thought.
  3 Flight of ideas.
VI   **Psychotic features of mania**:
  1 Delusions:
     (a) Grandiose delusions, e.g. the patient may believe that he is a religious prophet.
     (b) Persecutory delusions, e.g. the patient may believe that other people are conspiring against him because of his special importance.
     (c) Delusions of reference, e.g. the patient may believe that a remark heard on television is directed specifically to him (i.e. has a personal significance for him).
  2 Hallucinations:
     (a) Usually second person auditory hallucinations – taking the form of voices speaking to the patient about his special powers and consistent with the mood.
     (b) A few patients experience visual hallucinations, sometimes with a religious content.
VII **Cognition** – impaired attention and concentration – patient easily drawn to irrelevancies.
VIII **Insight** – invariably impaired – patient seldom thinks himself ill or in need of treatment.
IX   **Other psychiatric symptoms** – Schneiderian first-rank symptoms of schizophrenia – occur in 10–20% of manic patients.

Aetiology

I   **Genetic** – strong evidence for genetic aetiology provided by:
  1 Family studies – prevalence rate in first-degree relatives of patients with bipolar affective disorders is 15–20%. Prevalence rate in first-degree relatives of patients with unipolar affective disorders is 10–15%; cf. prevalence rate in general population of 5%.
  2 Twin studies:
     (a) Bipolar affective disorders – concordance rate in MZ twins is 79%; cf. 19% in DZ twins.
     (b) Unipolar affective disorders – concordance rate in MZ twins is 54%; cf. 20% in DZ twins.

II   Biochemical theories:
1   The monoamine theory of depression – depressive disorders are due to depletion, and mania to excessive provision, of a monoamine neurotransmitter at one or more sites in the brain.
Evidence for this theory:
(a)   Reserpine depletes presynaptic vesicles of monoamine stores and can result in depression.
(b)   Amphetamines cause the release of monoamines into the synaptic cleft and can result in euphoria.
(c)   Monoamine oxidase inhibitors (MAOIs) and monoamine re-uptake inhibitors (tricyclic antidepressants) increase the availability of monoamines to postsynaptic receptors and can elevate mood.
(d)   Post-mortem studies indicate decreased serotonin turnover in depression.
(e)   CSF (cerebrospinal fluid) and urinary studies indicate decreased levels of the breakdown products of noradrenaline and serotonin in some depressed patients.
2   Endocrine abnormalities:
(a)   Hypersecretion of cortisol in some depressives.
(b)   Decreased thyroid stimulating hormone (TSH) and growth hormone (GH) responses.
3   Electrolyte disturbances:
(a)   Intracellular ('residual') sodium increased in depression, further increased in mania.
(b)   Changes in erythrocyte membrane sodium–potassium ATPase – active transport of sodium and potassium increases on recovery from mania and depressive disorders.

III   Psychological theories:
1   Maternal deprivation – deprivation of maternal affection through separation or loss predisposes to depressive disorders in adult life.
2   Relationships with parents – patients with mild depressive disorders remember their parents as having been less caring and more over-protective, cf. patients with severe depressive disorders and normal controls.
3   Psychoanalytic theory:
(a)   Freud:
(i)   Depression thought to occur when feelings of love and hostility are present at the same time (ambivalence).
(ii)   The depressed patient regresses to the oral stage of psycho-sexual development, at which sadistic feelings are powerful.
(b)   Klein – if the child does not pass through the 'depressive position' successfully, he will be more likely to develop depression in adult life. The 'depressive position' is the stage of learning where

the infant acquires confidence that, when his mother leaves him, she will return even when he has been angry.

    (c)   Psychodynamic theory – mania is a defence against depression.

4   Cognitive theory – Beck suggests that a person who habitually adopts ways of thinking with depressive 'cognitive distortions' will be more likely to become depressed when faced with minor problems. There are four basic types of error shown by cognitive distortions in the cognitive theory of depression:

    (a)   Arbitrary inference – drawing a conclusion when there is no evidence for it and even some against it.

    (b)   Selective abstraction – focusing on a detail and ignoring more important features of a situation.

    (c)   Over-generalisation – drawing a general conclusion on the basis of a single incident.

    (d)   Minimisation and magnification – performance is underestimated and errors are overestimated.

5   Learned helplessness – depression results when highly desirable outcomes are believed improbable or highly aversive outcomes are believed probable, and the individual expects that no response of his will change their likelihood.

6   Separation experiments in animals – arise from the suggestion that the loss of a loved person may be a cause of depressive disorders. The studies may be of some importance to understanding the effects of separating human infants from their mothers.

7   Premorbid personality:

    (a)   Bipolar affective disorders – associated with cyclothymic personality traits (i.e. repeated and sustained mood swings).

    (b)   Unipolar affective disorders – associated with anankastic personality traits and readiness to develop anxiety.

IV   **Sociological theory** – In Brown's study (1975) of working-class women from inner London boroughs, the vulnerability factors for depression were:

1   Three or more children under 15 years of age at home.

2   Not working outside the home.

3   Lack of a supportive relationship with husband.

4   Loss of mother by death or separation before the age of 11.

5   An excess of threatening life events or major difficulties prior to the onset of depression.

V   **Life event studies** – depressives experience more life events (e.g. bereavement, separation) over normal controls in the six months prior to the onset of the disorder (Paykel, 1969).

VI   **Body build (Kretschmer)** – patients of pyknic (stocky and rounded) build are particularly prone to affective disorders.

Differential diagnosis

I   **Depressive disorders** – Exclude:
1   Neurotic disorders.
2   Schizophrenia.
3   Organic disorders – dementia, hypothyroidism.
II **Mania** – Exclude:
1   Schizophrenia.
2   Organic disorders – frontal lobe tumour, general paralysis of the insane (GPI), drug abuse.

Management

Physical

Antidepressants – used in the treatment of unipolar depression; can increase the frequency of cycling when used in bipolar affective disorder and therefore care needs to be taken when using them in bipolar disease.

I   TRICYCLIC ANTIDEPRESSANTS (TCAs)
A   IN GENERAL
   (a) **Mode of action**
      Monoamine re-uptake inhibitors (MARIs) – inhibit the re-uptake of both serotonin and noradrenaline into the presynaptic neurone, with the result that both neurotransmitters accumulate within the synapse. Such biochemical changes occur within several hours following administration of the drug, while the antidepressant action of the drug is delayed for about two weeks, indicating that some secondary process must be taking place.
   (b) **Indications**
      (i)   Treatment of depressive disorders in the acute stage.
      (ii)   Preventing relapse of depressive disorders.
      NB:
         (i) For the last decade or so, the generally held view among informed psychiatrists has been that 'the dose that gets you well is the dose that keeps you well'.
         (ii) TCAs are safer to use in pregnancy where the effects are more clearly established, cf. the more recently introduced antidepressants (SSRIs, SNRIs, noradrenergic and specific

serotonergic antidepressants [NaSSAs] and noradrenaline re-uptake inhibitors [NARIs]).

(iii) Antidepressants are non-addictive but are associated with a discontinuation syndrome – therefore they should be gradually withdrawn over a period of four weeks (when on the maximum dose), to minimise the risk of discontinuation symptoms.

(c) Adverse effects

1   Anticholinergic side-effects:
   (i)   Dry mouth.
   (ii)   Blurred vision.
   (iii)   Constipation.
   (iv)   Urinary retention.
   (v)   Tachycardia.
   (vi)   Impotence.
   (vii)   Sweating.
   (viii) Confusion.
   (ix)   Exacerbation of narrow angle glaucoma.

2   Cardiovascular side-effects (due to quinidine-like actions):
   (i)   Tachycardia.
   (ii)   Arrhythmias.
   (iii)   Postural hypotension.
   (iv)   Syncope.
   (v)   Cardiomyopathy.
   (vi)   Cardiac failure.
   (vii)   ECG changes (e.g. inversion and flattening of T waves).

3   Other side-effects:
   (i)   Seizures (due to lowering of the convulsive threshold).
   (ii)   Hypomania (in patients with bipolar affective disorder).
   (iii)   Tremor.
   (iv)   Weight gain.
   (v)   Agranulocytosis (uncommon).
   (vi)   Neuroleplic malignant syndrome (NMS) (rare).
   (vii)   Tardive dyskinesia (rare).

(d) Toxic effects (i.e. effects of overdosage)

1   Cardiac arrhythmias/arrest.
2   Prolongation of the QT interval.
3   Postural hypotension.
4   Epileptic seizures.
5   Hyperreflexia.
6   Mydriasis.
7   Coma.
8   Death.

B   MORE SPECIFICALLY

1   *Amitriptyline*

   (a) **Indications**

      Treatment of agitated depression – in view of its sedative nature:

      (i)   Starting dose – 75 mg nocte; build up gradually over 1–2 weeks to 150 mg nocte (usual dose required for efficacy in treating both the acute stage and for prophylaxis).

      (ii) In patients unresponsive to 150 mg nocte – pushing the dose up to 225 mg nocte or even 300 mg nocte (maximum) may be clinically effective; this would require ECG monitoring, as it is above the BNF (British National Formulary) maximum recommended dose (200 mg nocte).

   (b) **Adverse effects**

      Less suitable for the treatment of retarded depression – since it may exacerbate psychomotor retardation in such patients in view of its sedative nature.

2   *Imipramine*

   (a) **Indications**

      Treatment of retarded depression – in view of its alerting nature (similar dosage requirements as for amitriptyline – *see* earlier).

   (b) **Adverse effects**

      Less suitable for the treatment of agitated depression – since it may cause over-excitement in such patients in view of its alerting nature.

3   *Dosulepin (formerly known as dothiepin)*

   (a) **Indication**

      Treatment of agitated depression – in view of its sedative nature:

      (i)   Starting dose – 75 mg nocte, increased after four days to 150 mg nocte.

      (ii) In patients unresponsive to 150 mg nocte – pushing the dose up to 225 mg nocte may be clinically effective.

      (iii) Particularly useful in treating elderly patients – since it has fewer anticholinergic side-effects and fewer cardiovascular side-effects – cf. amitriptyline (this also explains why the starting dose of dosulepin can be stepped up more quickly to the therapeutic dose – cf. amitriptyline).

   (b) **Adverse effects**

      If taken in overdosage, dosulepin is the TCA most commonly responsible for deaths in the UK at present.

4   *Trazodone*
(a)   **Mode of action**
An antidepressant drug related to the TCAs – but a more selective inhibitor of the re-uptake of serotonin, cf. amitriptyline and imipramine.
(b)   **Indication**
Treatment of agitated depression – in view of its sedative nature:
(i)   Starting dose – 150 mg nocte.
(ii)   May be increased to 300 mg daily.
(iii)   Maximum dose of 600 mg daily in divided doses in hospitalised patients (in adults).
(c)   **Adverse effects**
(i)   Fewer anticholinergic side-effects and fewer cardiovascular side-effects, cf. amitriptyline.
(ii)   Safer in overdosage, cf. dosulepin.
(iii)   Rarely priapism (discontinue immediately).
5   *Clomipramine*
(a)   **Mode of action**
Inhibits the re-uptake of both serotonin and noradrenaline. However, it is a more selective inhibitor of the re-uptake of serotonin, cf. the other TCAs.
(b)   **Indication**
Treatment of agitated depression – in view of its sedative nature.
(c)   **Adverse effects**
It has more anticholinergic side-effects and more cardiovascular side-effects – cf. amitriptyline – which may prevent some patients from tolerating it.

II   **MONOAMINE OXIDASE INHIBITORS (MAOIs)**
(a)   **Mode of action**
Inhibit the enzyme monoamine oxidase which is present in the presynaptic neurone and provides an important pathway for the metabolism of monoamines; thus, MAOIs inhibit the intraneuronal metabolism of monoamines, resulting in enhanced release of amine neurotransmitters into the synapse.
(b)   **Indications**
(i)   Treatment of atypical depressive disorders with anxiety, phobic anxiety, obsessional, dissociative (conversion) or hypochondriacal symptoms.
(ii)   Treatment of resistant depression (particularly tranylcypromine – but it carries a risk of dependence because of its amphetamine-like action).

(c) **Adverse effects**
  (i) Potentiate the pressor effect of tyramine and dopa present in certain foods (e.g. Chianti wine, cheese spreads, well-hung game, pickled herring, banana skins, broad bean 'pods', Marmite and Bovril).
  (ii) Potentiate the pressor effect of indirect-acting sympathomimetic drugs (e.g. proprietary cough mixtures, nasal decongestants, anaesthetics).

  NB: Both of these types of interaction may cause a dangerous rise in blood pressure ('hypertensive crisis') with fatal consequences; an early warning sign may be a throbbing headache.

  (iii) TCAs, second-generation antidepressants and SSRIs should not be started until two weeks after MAOIs have been stopped in view of the persistence of the effects of MAOIs following discontinuation.
  (iv) MAOIs should not be started until one week after TCAs and second-generation antidepressants have been stopped.
  (v) MAOIs should not be started until two weeks after SSRIs have been stopped with the exception of fluoxetine (*see* below).
  (vi) MAOIs should not be started until five weeks after fluoxetine has been stopped in view of its long half-life and active metabolite (norfluoxetine).
  (vii) The most commonly prescribed MAOI is phenelzine; however, MAOIs are the least commonly prescribed of the antidepressant drugs because:
    (a) They interact dangerously with certain foods and drugs (*see* above).
    (b) The washout period following MAOI discontinuation is two weeks – cf. the washout period of one week following discontinuation of TCAs and second-generation antidepressants (*see* above).
    (c) The main indication for MAOIs is atypical depressive disorders (*see* above), i.e. MAOIs are not generally indicated for endogenous depressive disorders with biological features of depression (except resistant cases when they may be combined with TCAs under specialist supervision).

III **REVERSIBLE INHIBITORS OF MONOAMINE OXIDASE TYPE A (RIMAs)**
Moclobemide (the first RIMA) was introduced into the UK in 1993.
(a) **Mode of action**
  Selectively and reversibly inhibits monoamine oxidase type A. In contrast, conventional MAOIs inhibit monoamine oxidase types A and B and are irreversible.

The antidepressant effect of MAOIs is considered to be a result of inhibition of monoamine oxidase type A.

(b) **Indications**

  (i)   Treatment of endogenous and atypical depressive disorders (dosage: 150–600 mg daily in divided doses; however, there are anecdotal reports of higher doses required for efficacy in endogenous depressive disorders).

  (ii) Treatment of resistant depression (particularly when the patient is unwilling to try a conventional MAOI).

(c) **Adverse effects**

  (i)   Claimed to cause less potentiation of the pressor effect of tyramine and dopa-containing foods, cf. conventional MAOIs – however, patients should still avoid consuming large amounts of such foods.

  (ii) Claimed to cause less potentiation of the pressor effect of indirect-acting sympathomimetic drugs, cf. conventional MAOIs – however, patients should still avoid such drugs.

  (iii) No treatment-free washout period is required after it has been stopped in view of its short duration of action, cf. conventional MAOIs.

  (iv) Should not be started until one week after TCAs, second-generation antidepressants and conventional MAOIs have been stopped.

  (v)   Should not be started until two weeks after SSRIs have been stopped with the exception of fluoxetine (*see* below).

  (vi) Should not be started until five weeks after fluoxetine has been stopped.

  (vii) Contraindicated in agitated or excited patients – an unfortunate adverse effect since the majority of clinically depressed patients present this way.

  (viii) May precipitate hypomania in patients with bipolar affective disorder.

  (ix) May be the antidepressant of choice in patients with epilepsy.

IV SECOND-GENERATION ANTIDEPRESSANTS

A   IN GENERAL

(a) **Definition**

The next class of antidepressant drugs to be developed after TCAs.

(b) **Indications**

Particularly useful in the following groups of depressed patients:

  (i)   Patients intolerant of the side-effects of TCAs.

  (ii) Elderly patients.

      (iii) Patients at high risk of suicide.

      (iv) Patients treated in the general practice setting.

  (c) **Adverse effects**

      (i)   Fewer anticholinergic side-effects and fewer cardiovascular side-effects – cf. TCAs.

      (ii) Safer in overdosage – cf. TCAs.

B   MORE SPECIFICALLY

1   *Lofepramine*

  (a) **Mode of action**

      (i)   Mainly a noradrenergic re-uptake inhibitor, i.e. it is a relatively selective re-uptake inhibitor of noradrenaline.

      (ii) Structurally a tricyclic antidepressant – however, its adverse effects profile is considerably different from the older 'parent' TCAs (*see* below).

  (b) **Indication**

      Treatment and prophylaxis of retarded depression – in view of its alerting nature (dosage: 70 mg b.d.; this may be increased to 70 mg mane, 140 mg nocte).

  (c) **Adverse effects**

      (i)   Less suitable for the treatment of agitated depression – since it may cause over-excitement (e.g. sweating, palpitations) in such patients in view of its alerting nature.

      (ii) Much improved side-effects profile – cf. older 'parent' TCAs – i.e. lofepramine has fewer anticholinergic side-effects and less cardiotoxicity. Hence, more suitable for use in physically ill patients, cf. older 'parent' TCAs.

      (iii) Remarkable record of safety in overdosage – only three deaths recorded to date.

      (iv) May be the antidepressant of choice in pregnancy.

2   *Mianserin*

  (a) **Mode of action**

      (i)   An α_2 presynaptic autoreceptor antagonist – a novel mode of action for an antidepressant drug with no significant effect on the re-uptake of monoamines (i.e. it is only a weak inhibitor of serotonin and noradrenaline re-uptake); despite this, it still appears to be an effective antidepressant.

      (ii) Structurally a tetracyclic antidepressant.

  (b) **Adverse effects**

      (i)   No anticholinergic side-effects.

      (ii) Minimal cardiotoxicity – safer in overdosage.   } cf. TCAs

      (iii) Rarely causes convulsions – i.e. less pro-convulsive.

(iv) May cause agranulocytosis (particularly in the elderly):
- a full blood count is recommended every four weeks during the first three months of treatment.
- if signs of infection develop (e.g. sore throat, fever, stomatitis), treatment should be stopped, a full blood count obtained and subsequent clinical monitoring should continue.
- this unfortunate side-effect of mianserin together with its questionable efficacy (*see* mode of action earlier) has limited the prescription of the drug in the hospital setting.

V SELECTIVE SEROTONIN RE-UPTAKE INHIBITORS (SSRIs) (ALSO KNOWN AS 5-HT RE-UPTAKE INHIBITORS)
A IN GENERAL
(a) **Definition**
The next class of antidepressant drugs to follow the second-generation antidepressants in time, i.e. SSRIs, are effectively 'third generation antidepressants'.

(b) **Mode of action**
SSRIs are highly selective serotonin re-uptake inhibitors with little or no effect on noradrenergic processes.

(c) **Indications**
1 Treatment of depressive disorders, particularly in:
(i) Patients intolerant of the side-effects of TCAs.
(ii) Elderly patients.
(iii) Patients with a high risk of suicide.
(iv) Patients treated in the general practice setting.
(v) Patients with cardiovascular disease.
2 Preventing relapse of depressive disorders – need to continue medication for six months postclinical recovery after the first episode of a unipolar affective disorder and for several (one to three) years postclinical recovery after two or more episodes of a unipolar affective disorder.
NB: If patient fails to respond to one SSRI after an adequate trial (i.e. 4–6 weeks at the maximum dose), there is a tendency to try one other SSRI before switching to a different class of antidepressant.

(d) **Adverse effects**
(i) No anticholinergic side-effects.
(ii) No clinically significant cardiovascular side-effects.
(iii) More gastrointestinal side-effects (e.g. nausea, vomiting, diarrhoea) which are dose-related.
(iv) More sexual dysfunction (e.g. delayed ejaculation in men, anorgasmia in women).
(v) Safer in overdosage.

cf. TCAs

(vi)   In keeping with good clinical practice, SSRIs should be with-drawn slowly to minimise the risk of discontinuation symp-toms.

(vii)   Inhibition of the liver enzyme cytochrome P4502D6, which is responsible for metabolising the SSRIs and other drugs that might be coprescribed. There is little convincing evidence of clinically significant drug interactions.

(viii) No clinically significant interaction with alcohol – therefore SSRIs may be prescribed to patients comorbid for alcohol problems and clinical depression.

(ix)   May be less likely to precipitate hypomania in patients with bipolar affective disorder, cf. TCAs.

(x)   May only be prescribed at a therapeutic dose, cf. TCAs which have tended to be prescribed at a subtherapeutic dose in the general practice setting.

(xi)   Less likely to cause weight gain, cf. TCAs.

(xii)   Extra-pyramidal side-effects (EPSE) (including akathisia) are reported to the Committee on Safety of Medicines (CSM).

B   MORE SPECIFICALLY

1   *Fluvoxamine*

The first SSRI introduced into the UK in 1987.

(a) **Mode of action**

   (i)   Structurally a monocyclic antidepressant.
   (ii)   No active metabolite.
   (iii) 17–22 hour half-life.

(b) **Indication**

   Treatment of depression (starting dose 50 mg nocte to 100 mg nocte; dose range: 50 mg o.d. to 150 mg b.d.)

(c) **Adverse effects**

   (i)   High incidence of nausea and vomiting particularly during the first few days of treatment – this may prevent some patients from tolerating it; such gastrointestinal side-effects may be offset somewhat by taking tablets immediately after food and by initiating treatment at a dosage of 50 mg nocte for one week and then stepping it up to the usual therapeutic dosage of 50 mg b.d. (some patients may only respond to the higher therapeutic dosage of 100 mg b.d. or the even higher dosage of 150 mg b.d.).

   (ii)   Less suitable for patients with hepatic impairment – since it may elevate hepatic enzymes with symptoms.

   (iii) Increases the plasma concentration of theophylline.

2   *Fluoxetine*
    Introduced into the UK in 1989.
    (a) **Mode of action**
        (i)   Structurally a bicyclic antidepressant.
        (ii) Long half-life (2–4 days with an active metabolite (norfluoxetine) which itself has a long half-life with similar activity to the parent compound.
    (b) **Indication**
        Treatment of depression (dosage: 20 mg mane; this may be increased up to 80 mg mane in adults by gradual 20 mg increments if necessary).
    (c) **Adverse effects**
        (i)   Less suitable for the treatment of agitated depression – since it may cause over-excitement (e.g. restlessness, nervousness) in such patients in view of its alerting nature.
        (ii) Less suitable for patients with severe renal impairment – in view of its long half-life and active metabolite.
        (iii) Less suitable for patients with severe weight loss – in view of its catabolic/anorectic nature.
        (iv) Nausea and vomiting appear to be less of a problem with fluoxetine, cf. fluvoxamine.
        (v)   Increases the plasma concentration of the antiarrhythmic flecainide by cytochrome P4502D6 inhibition.
        (vi) Other significant drug interactions – increases the plasma concentration of:
              – Haloperidol.
              – Clozapine.
              – TCAs.
              – Phenytoin.
              – Warfarin.

3   *Sertraline*
    Introduced into the UK in 1990.
    (a) **Mode of action**
        (i)   Structurally different from fluvoxamine, fluoxetine and paroxetine.
        (ii) Has an active metabolite (desmethylsertraline) which has a long half-life with about one-eighth of the activity of the parent compound.
    (b) **Indications**
        (i)   Treatment of depression (dose range: 50 mg mane to 200 mg mane).
        (ii) Prevention of relapse in depression and recurrent depression.

(c) **Adverse effects**
   (i)   Side-effects include loose stools and diarrhoea.
   (ii) May be the antidepressant of choice in patients with renal impairment.
   (iii) May have lower potential for drug interactions – since it has no significant interaction with cytochrome P4502D6.

4   *Paroxetine*
Introduced into the UK in 1991.
   (a) **Mode of action**
      (i)   Structurally different from fluvoxamine, fluoxetine and sertraline.
      (ii) No active metabolite.
      (iii) 24-hour half-life.
   (b) **Indications**
      (i)   Treatment of depression with associated anxiety – the first SSRI to have a licence for this (dosage: 20 mg mane; this may be increased up to 50 mg daily in adults by gradual 10 mg increments if necessary).
      (ii) Prevention of relapse in depression.
   (c) **Adverse effects**
      (i)   Less suitable for the treatment of retarded (anergic) depression – in view of its anxiolytic nature.
      (ii) Nausea and vomiting appear to be less of a problem with paroxetine, cf. fluvoxamine.
      (iii) Inhibits its own metabolism by cytochrome P4502D6 inhibition.
      (iv) Side-effects include a dry mouth and drowsiness.
      (v)   When discontinuing paroxetine, it should be gradually reduced by weekly 10 mg increments to minimise the risk of discontinuation symptoms, i.e. when on the maximum dose of 50 mg daily in adults for depression, this should be gradually withdrawn over a period of four weeks.

5   *Citalopram*
Introduced into the UK in 1995.
   (a) **Mode of action**
      (i)   Structurally different from the other SSRIs.
      (ii) No active metabolite.
   (b) **Indications**
      (i)   Treatment of depression (dosage: 20 mg daily; this may be increased up to 60 mg daily in adults by gradual 20 mg increments if necessary).
      (ii) Prevention of relapse in depression and recurrent depression.

(c) **Adverse effects**
    (i)   May have lower potential for drug interactions – since it has no significant interaction with cytochrome P4502D6.

6   *Escitalopram*
Introduced into the UK in 2002.
(a) **Mode of action**
    (i)   The S-enantiomer of citalopram, i.e. the optical isomer of citalopram with antidepressant activity.
    (ii)   More selective than citalopram – which consists of the racemic mixture of both the S-enantiomer and the R-enantiomer (the latter lacks antidepressant activity).
    (iii) Serotonin transporter theory:
           – By removing R-citalopram (at the synapse), escitalopram functions more effectively.
           – Escitalopram increases serotonin levels more than citalopram.
(b) **Indications**
    (i)   Treatment of depression (dosage: 10 mg daily; this may be increased up to 20 mg daily in adults).
    (ii)   May be associated with an early symptom relief.
    (iii) Some evidence that efficacy is comparable to venlafaxine XL, cf. other SSRIs where there is considerable evidence that venlafaxine XL is more effective.
(c) **Adverse effects**
    (i)   Escitalopram has a comparable side-effect profile to citalopram.
    (ii)   Co-administration with the known cytochrome P450 isoenzyme CYP2C19 inhibitors omeprazole and high dose cimetidine, may require reduction of the escitalopram dose (metabolism of escitalopram is mainly mediated by CYP2C19).

VI SEROTONIN AND NORADRENALINE RE-UPTAKE INHIBITORS (SNRIs)

1   *Venlafaxine*
The first SNRI introduced into the UK in 1995. Available as a standard formulation requiring twice-daily dosing (up to 375 mg daily) and a modified release formulation (XL) to allow once-daily dosing (up to 225 mg daily)
(a) **Mode of action**
    (i)   Structurally a bicyclic antidepressant.

(ii) It selectively inhibits the re-uptake of both serotonin and noradrenaline into the presynaptic neurone (but the predominant effect is on serotonin):

– At low dose (75 mg daily), its predominant action is on serotonin inhibition, with a lesser action on noradrenaline inhibition.

– At moderate dose to high dose, it acts more equally as both a serotonin and noradrenaline re-uptake inhibitor.

(b) Indications

(i) Treatment of depressive disorders (dosage: 75 mg daily; this may be increased to 150 mg daily in moderate-to-severe depression and again if necessary to the maximum dose of 225 mg daily for the XL formulation; it may be further increased by 75 mg increments every 2–3 days to a maximum of 375 mg daily in hospitalised severe depression – this would require twice-daily dosing of the standard formulation).

(ii) There is now considerable evidence that venlafaxine XL is more effective than the SSRIs; however, there is some evidence that the efficacy of escitalopram is comparable to venlafaxine XL.

(iii) Some evidence for treatment of resistant depression – either as monotherapy or augmented with a mood stabiliser, cf. combining it with another antidepressant (as it has a dual action on serotonin and adrenaline).

(c) Adverse effects

(i) Fewer anticholinergic side-effects.

(ii) Fewer sedative side-effects.   } cf. TCAs

(iii) Safer in overdosage.

(iv) Less likely to cause weight gain.

(v) Gastrointestinal side-effects (e.g. nausea) – these are dose related and occur with a similar prevalence to those observed with SSRIs; they appear to be reduced with the XL formulation.

(vi) Blood pressure should be monitored in patients taking 75 mg daily or more.

(vii) May precipitate hypomania in patients with bipolar affective disorder.

(viii) Frequently reported side-effects are sweating and headache.

(ix) Drug interactions – potentiation of the anticoagulant effects of warfarin has been reported.

(x) Should not be used in patients with pre-existing heart disease.

(xi) Should not be used in patients with pre-existing untreated or uncontrolled hypertension.

(xii) New patients should have a baseline ECG and blood pressure measurement.

(xiii) Should only be initiated by specialist mental health practitioners (including GPs with a special interest in mental
health).

2   *Duloxetine*

Introduced into the UK in 2005.

(a) **Mode of action**

(i) It selectively inhibits the re-uptake of both serotonin and
noradrenaline into the presynaptic neurone. It is a relatively
balanced inhibitor of both neurotransmitters, cf. venlafaxine
where at low dose (75 mg daily), its predominant action is
on serotonin inhibition, with a lesser action on noradrenaline
inhibition.

NB: *Clinical benefits cannot be inferred from pre-clinical binding studies.*

(ii) It has no significant affinity for dopaminergic, adrenergic,
muscarinic or histaminergic receptors.

(b) **Indications**

(i) Treatment of depressive disorders (dosage: starting and maintenance dose of 60 mg daily; this may be increased to a maximum dose of 60 mg b.d. – however, there is no clinical evidence
suggesting that patients not responding to 60 mg daily may
benefit from dose up-titrations).

(ii) Provides relief across a broad range of depressive symptoms
(both psychological and somatic).

(iii) Helps to relieve the general aches and pains (GAPs) seen in
depressed patients including back pain and shoulder pain.

(c) **Adverse effects**

(i) Most commonly reported adverse effects are nausea, dry mouth
and constipation; of the commonly reported adverse effects, the
majority are mild-to-moderate and transient.

(ii) No clinically significant effect on weight.

(iii) Blood pressure monitoring is recommended as appropriate in
patients with pre-existing heart disease and/or pre-existing
hypertension, cf. venlafaxine which should not be used in patients
with pre-existing heart disease and/or pre-existing untreated or
uncontrolled hypertension.

(iv) No clinically significant prolongation of the QT_C interval, cf.
venlafaxine where new patients should have a baseline ECG.

(v) May be initiated by GPs, cf. venlafaxine which should only be
initiated by specialist mental health practitioners (including GPs
with a special interest in mental health).

(vi) Contraindications:
– Hepatic impairment/severe renal impairment.
– MAOIs.

- The known cytochrome P450 isoenzyme CYP1A2 inhibitor fluvoxamine.
(vii) Cautions:
- Bipolar affective disorder/seizures.
- Other SSRIs/TCAs/venlafaxine.
- Warfarin.
- Products that are predominantly metabolised by cytochrome P4502D6 if they have a narrow therapeutic index.
(viii) In keeping with good clinical practice, duloxetine should be withdrawn slowly to minimise the risk of discontinuation symptoms.

NB: The contrasts with venlafaxine are based on the summary of product characteristics (SPC), cf. head to head trial data.

The SPC for duloxetine is based on the clinical trial population at present – although the data set is quite large, it is still not based on naturalistic findings, which will only come out once duloxetine has been on the market for a while, cf. venlafaxine, which has been on the market for a long time so much more data has accrued.

VII NORADRENERGIC AND SPECIFIC SEROTONERGIC ANTIDEPRESSANTS (NaSSAs)

Mirtazapine (the first NaSSA) was launched in the UK in 1997 as a conventional tablet. This was phased out by 4th May 2004.

The world's first ever antidepressant available as an orally disintegrating tablet – launched in the UK in 2003. This soltab formulation should be placed on the tongue and allowed to dissolve, i.e. melt.

(a) **Mode of action**
  (i)   A presynaptic α_2-autoreceptor antagonist – thus enhancing noradrenergic neurotransmission (like mianserin).
  (ii)   A presynaptic α_2-heteroreceptor antagonist – thus preventing the inhibitory effect of noradrenaline on serotonin receptors.
  (iii) A postsynaptic serotonin $5HT_2$- and $5HT_3$-receptor antagonist – thus enhancing serotonergic neurotransmission specifically via $5HT_1$- postsynaptic receptors.
  (iv)   No significant effect on the re-uptake of monoamines, cf. TCAs, SSRIs, SNRIs and NARIs (*see* next section).
  (v)   A postsynaptic histamine H_1-receptor antagonist.
  (vi)   It has a dual action on both serotonin and noradrenaline from the starting dose (30 mg).

(b) **Indications**
- (i) Treatment of depressive disorders (dosage: 30 mg nocte; this may be increased to 45 mg nocte if further clinical improvement is required or if oversedation occurs; it may be decreased to 15 mg nocte if further sedation is required).

  NB: Mirtazapine becomes more sedative as the dosage is decreased due to its antihistaminergic effect predominating over its noradrenergic effect. Conversely, it becomes less sedative as the dosage is increased due to its noradrenergic effect predominating over its antihistaminergic effect.
- (ii) Some evidence for treatment of resistant depression in combination with an SSRI – if there has been a partial response to the SSRI alone after an adequate trial (4–6 weeks at the maximum dosage).

(c) **Adverse effects**
- (i) Significantly higher incidence of weight gain, cf. placebo – which may be partially due to increased appetite.
- (ii) Significantly higher incidence of drowsiness and excessive sedation, cf. placebo – owing to a strong affinity for histamine H_1-receptors.
- (iii) May lack some serotonin-related side-effects – possibly owing to the blockade of serotonin $5HT_2$-receptors which mediate sexual dysfunction/insomnia/agitation/anxiety and blockade of serotonin $5HT_3$-receptors which mediate nausea/vomiting/headache.
- (iv) Lacks cardiovascular side-effects – owing to a very low affinity for α_1-adrenergic receptors.
- (v) Lacks anticholinergic side-effects – owing to a very low affinity for muscarinic receptors.
- (vi) Blood pressure monitoring is not required, cf. venlafaxine XL.
- (vii) There is no clinically significant interaction with warfarin, cf. venlafaxine XL.
- (viii) When switching antidepressants, the novel action of mirtazapine reduces the risks of the serotonin syndrome.
- (ix) When switching antidepressants, there is no washout period usually required with mirtazapine, so patient therapy is not interrupted (except for MAOIs).

VIII NORADRENALINE RE-UPTAKE INHIBITORS (NARIs)

Reboxetine (the first NARI) was launched in the UK in 1997.

(a) **Mode of action**

A highly selective noradrenaline re-uptake inhibitor with no significant effect on serotonergic processes.

(b) **Indications**
   (i) Treatment of depression (dosage: 4 mg b.d. in adults; if further clinical improvement is required, this may be increased to 6 mg mane, 4 mg nocte and again if necessary to the maximum dosage of 6 mg b.d. in adults).
(c) **Adverse effects**
   (i) Anticholinergic side-effects (e.g. dry mouth, constipation).
   (ii) It is not recommended for use in the elderly.
   (iii) When switching antidepressants, the predominantly noradrenergic action of reboxetine reduces the risk of the serotonin syndrome.
   (iv) When switching antidepressants, there is no washout period usually required with reboxetine, so patient therapy is not interrupted (except for MAOIs).

IX   BUSPIRONE
(a) **Mode of action**
   (i) Thought to act at specific serotonin ($5HT_{1A}$) presynaptic autoreceptors – as a partial agonist.
   (ii) Response to treatment may take up to two weeks – similar to antidepressant drugs.
(b) **Indications**
   (i) May be useful in the treatment of resistant depression – as an augmenting agent to SSRIs (by enhancing serotonin accumulation within the synapse).
(c) **Adverse effects**
   (i) Physical dependence and abuse liability low.
   (ii) Non-toxic augmenting agent, cf. lithium carbonate.

X   PINDOLOL
(a) **Indications***
   (i) Some evidence for treatment of resistant depression as an augmenting agent to SSRIs (by enhancing serotonergic accumulation within the synapse).
   (ii) Some evidence for treatment of resistant depression as part of the triple therapy:
       – SSRI.
       – Buspirone.
       – Pindolol.

XI   THYROXINE
(a) **Indications***
   (i) It may be used to augment antidepressant drug treatment in resistant depression.

* These indications are not currently licensed in the UK.

(ii)   It may have mood-elevating properties when clinical depression and subclinical hypothyroidism co-exist (the latter being defined as a free thyroxine serum level at the lower end of the normal range).

Mood stabilising drugs – used in the treatment of bipolar affective disorder

I   LITHIUM CARBONATE
   (a)   **Mode of action**
      The precise mechanism by which lithium produces its therapeutic effect is complex and poorly understood.
      Postulated mechanisms of therapeutic effects:
      (i)   Decreased neurotransmitter postsynaptic receptor sensitivity.
      (ii)   Stimulates exit of Na^+ from cells where intracellular Na^+ is elevated (as in depression) by stimulating the Na^+/K^+ pump mechanism.
      (iii)   Stimulates entry of Na^+ into cells where intracellular Na^+ is reduced (as in mania).
      (iv)   Influences Ca^{2+} and Na^+ transfer across cell membranes including the Ca^{2+}-dependent release of neurotransmitter.
      (v)   Inhibits both cyclic AMP and inositol phosphate 'second messenger' systems in the membrane – this mechanism mediates the long-term side-effects of nephrogenic diabetes insipidus and hypothyroidism (*see* below), i.e. lithium blocks ADH (antidiurelic hormone)-sensitive adenyl cyclase and TSH-sensitive adenyl cyclase, respectively.
      (vi)   Interacts with Ca^{2+} and Mg^{2+}, thereby increasing cell membrane permeability.
   (b)   **Indications**
   1   Treatment of depressive disorders:
      (i)   Treatment can be justified in the acute stages of depressive disorders, when other measures have failed.
      (ii)   Treatment of resistant depression – i.e. effective in patients who have failed to respond to a cyclic antidepressant drug (mono-, bi-, tri- or tetracyclic antidepressants).
      (iii)   Enhances the effects of TCAs and MAOIs.
      (iv)   Enhances the effects of SSRIs – however, lithium should be introduced cautiously because of the risk of the serotonin syndrome developing (owing to enhanced serotonergic activity); this risk appears to be lowest with fluvoxamine.

2   Preventing relapse of depressive disorders:
　　(i)　In unipolar affective disorders:
　　　　– Lithium reduces the rate of relapse (but is probably no more effective than continuing TCA treatment).
　　　　– After the first episode, treatment should be prolonged for six months postclinical recovery.
　　　　– After two or more episodes – treatment should be prolonged for several (1–3) years postclinical recovery; lithium is particularly useful in the prophylaxis of recurrent unipolar depression.
　　　　– Continuing treatment with lithium reduces the rate of relapse after treatment with ECT.
　　(ii)　In bipolar affective disorders – prolonged administration of lithium (five years) prevents relapses into depression.
3   Treatment of mania:
　　Lithium is effective in high doses (1000 mg nocte), but therapeutic response usually only occurs in the second week of treatment; thus, the response of lithium is slower than the response to antipsychotic drugs.
4   Preventing relapse of mania:
　　In bipolar affective disorders, prolonged administration of lithium (five years) prevents relapse into mania.
5   Treatment of mixed affective states.
(c)   **Adverse effects**
1   Short-term side-effects:
　　(i)　Gastrointestinal disturbances (nausea, vomiting, diarrhoea).
　　(ii)　Fine tremor.
　　(iii)　Muscle weakness.
　　(iv)　Polyuria.
　　(v)　Polydypsia.
2   Long-term side-effects:
　　(i)　Nephrogenic diabetes insipidus.
　　(ii)　Hypothyroidism.
　　(iii)　Cardiotoxicity.
　　(iv)　Irreversible renal damage (in patients with pre-existing renal pathology).
　　(v)　Oedema.
　　(vi)　Weight gain.
　　(vii)　Tardive dyskinesia and other movement disorders.
3   Toxic effects:
　　(i)　Increasing gastrointestinal disturbances (anorexia, vomiting, diarrhoea)

(ii)   Increasing CNS disturbances (coarse tremor, drowsiness, ataxia, nystagmus, incoordination, slurring of speech, convulsions, coma).

(iii)   The effects of lithium overdosage may be fatal – hence it is important that the serum lithium level be closely monitored to ensure that it lies within the therapeutic range of 0.4–1.0 mmol/l (the lower end of this range is for maintenance therapy; the higher end of this range is for treatment in the acute stages of illness) on blood samples taken 12 hours after the last dose of lithium; serum lithium levels over 1.5 mmol/l may be fatal.

(iv)   Once stabilised on lithium carbonate, the following should be monitored:
– Every 3 months – serum lithium level and serum urea and electrolytes.
– Every 6 months – thyroid functions test.
– Every 12 months – ECG.

NB: *Before commencing lithium therapy, baseline investigations should include a serum urea and electrolytes, a thyroid function test and an ECG.*

4   Drug interactions:

(i)   Sodium depletion raises the serum lithium level and may result in lithium toxicity – therefore the concurrent use of diuretics (particularly thiazides) should be avoided.

(ii)   The concurrent use of carbamazepine with lithium may result in neurotoxicity without raising the serum lithium level – hence if carbamazepine is added to lithium, it should be done so with caution – cf. the concurrent use of sodium valproate with lithium which is safe.

(iii)   NSAIDs raise the serum lithium level and may result in lithium toxicity – therefore their concurrent use with lithium should be avoided.

(iv)   ACE inhibitors raise the serum lithium level.

5   Contraindications

(i)   Pregnancy.

(ii)   Breast feeding.

(iii)   Renal impairment.

II CARBAMAZEPINE

Available as a standard formulation requiring three times a day dosing and a modified release formulation (Tegretol Retard) to allow twice-daily dosing (up to 800 mg b.d.).

(a) Mode of action

1   Structurally similar to the tricyclic antidepressant imipramine – however, carbamazepine has no effect on monoamine re-uptake.

2   Thought to mediate its therapeutic effect by inhibiting kindling phenomena in the limbic system.

(b) **Indications**

1   Treatment of depressive disorders:
   (i)   Treatment of resistant depression, i.e. worth a trial in patients who have failed to respond to a cyclic antidepressant drug and lithium carbonate.
   (ii)   Enhances the effects of TCAs and SSRIs.

2   Preventing relapse of depressive disorders:
   (i)   It prevents relapses into depression in both recurrent unipolar affective disorders and recurrent bipolar affective disorders.
   (ii)   It is the mood stabiliser of choice in patients with both epilepsy and bipolar affective disorder since it also has anticonvulsant properties.

3   Treatment of mania – carbamazepine is effective in high doses (600 mg b.d. to 800 mg b.d.), but the therapeutic response usually only occurs in the second week of treatment; thus, the response to carbamazepine is slower than the response to antipsychotic drugs.

4   Preventing relapse of mania:
   (i)   In patients who fail to respond to lithium carbonate – carbamazepine can either be substituted for, or added to, lithium; the two drugs appear to have a synergistic effect when used in combination (but *see* earlier note on their concurrent use).
   (ii)   In patients with the rapid-cycling form of bipolar affective disorder (i.e. four or more affective episodes per year) – carbamazepine is a better prophylactic agent than lithium carbonate.

(c) **Adverse effects**

1   Side-effects:
   (i)   Dizziness and drowsiness.
   (ii)   Generalised erythematous rash (3%).
   (iii) Visual disturbances (especially double vision).
   (iv)   Gastrointestinal disturbances (anorexia, constipation).
   (v)   Leucopenia and other blood disorders.
   (vi)   Hyponatraemia.

2   Carbamazepine must be initiated at a dosage of 200 mg b.d. (due to autoinduction, i.e. it often raises the serum level of an active metabolite of carbamazepine) and increased after one week to the usual therapeutic dosage of 200 mg mane, 400 mg nocte required for prophylaxis (some patients may require 400 mg b.d.) – carbamazepine is a less toxic drug than lithium carbonate and regular serum level estimation appears to be unnecessary; however, because of the slight risk of leucopenia and other blood disorders, it is important that full blood count is monitored periodically.

3   Carbamazepine is an inducer of the liver enzyme cytochrome P4502D6 – thus it can lower plasma haloperidol levels by half.
4   Carbamazepine also decreases the plasma concentration of:
     (i)   Oral contraceptives.
     (ii) Warfarin.
5   The plasma concentration of carbamazepine is increased by:
     (i)   Erythromycin.
     (ii) Cimetidine.
     (iii) Calcium-channel blockers.
     (iv) Isoniazid.
6   The plasma concentration of carbamazepine is reduced by:
        Phenytoin.
NB: *The maximum dosage of carbamazepine is 800 mg b.d. (prescribed as tegretol retard).*

III   SODIUM VALPROATE / VALPROATE SEMISODIUM

Sodium valproate is available as a standard formulation requiring three times a day dosing and a modified release formulation (Epilim Chrono) to allow twice-daily dosing (maximum of 2.5 g daily in divided doses).
NB: *Valproate semisodium (comprising equimolar amounts of sodium valproate and valproic acid) is currently licensed in the UK and USA for bipolar affective disorder. Sodium valproate has also been used, but it is unlicensed for this indication. In terms of cost, valproate semisodium is approximately five times more expensive than sodium valproate (prescribed as Epilim Chrono) for equivalent dosages.*

(a)   **Mode of action**
1   Sodium valproate is thought to mediate its therapeutic effect through indirect effects on gamma-aminobutyric acid (GABA)-ergic systems (i.e. it may slow GABA breakdown by inhibiting succinic semi-aldehyde dehydrogenase), implicating a possible underlying biochemical disturbance of GABA deficiency in some affective disorders.
2   Valproate semisodium is thought to permeate the blood–brain barrier more easily, cf. sodium valproate – this, in turn, results in a higher concentration of valproate in the brain with valproate semisodium, cf. an equivalent dose of sodium valproate.

(b)   **Indications**
1   Treatment of depressive disorders:
     (i)   Treatment of resistant depression, i.e. worth a trial in patients who have failed to respond to a cyclic antidepressant drug, lithium carbonate and carbamazepine.
     (ii) Enhances the effects of TCAs and SSRIs.
2   Preventing relapse of depressive disorders – it prevents relapses into depression in bipolar affective disorders.

3   Treatment of mania – sodium valproate is effective in high doses (600 mg b.d. to 1200 mg b.d.), but the therapeutic response usually only occurs in the second week of treatment; thus, the response to sodium valproate is slower than the response to antipsychotic drugs.

NB: *With semisodium valproate, the therapeutic response is claimed to occur in the first week of treatment, cf. sodium valproate [the dosing for valproate semisodium is 750 mg daily in divided doses (day one), then 500 mg b.d. to 1000 mg b.d. or 20 mg/kg/day from day two onwards].*

4   Preventing relapse of mania:
   (i)   Effective as a mood stabiliser in some manic patients who fail to respond to lithium carbonate and carbamazepine.
   (ii)   In the case of lithium carbonate, sodium valproate can be safely added to it and has been shown to enhance the effectiveness of lithium as a mood stabiliser.
   (iii) May also be used as a first-line treatment – on both clinical and litigation grounds, valproate semisodium should be preferred to sodium valproate.

NB: *It is better to prescribe valproate semisodium as the brand Depakote, to avoid confusion with sodium valproate.*

(c) **Adverse effects**

1   Side-effects
   (i)   Recent concern over severe hepatic and pancreatic toxicity.
   (ii)   Haematological disturbance (thrombocytopenia, inhibition of platelet aggregation).
   (iii) Drowsiness, weight gain and hair loss.

2   Sodium valproate is initiated at a dosage of 200 mg b.d. and increased after one week to 400 mg b.d. and again after another week to 600 mg b.d., the usual therapeutic dosage required for prophylaxis (some patients may require 800 mg b.d.) – sodium valproate is a less toxic drug than lithium and regular serum level estimation appears to be unnecessary; however, because of the slight risk of severe hepatic toxicity, severe pancreatic toxicity and haematological disturbance of platelet function, it is important that liver function tests, serum amylase level and full blood count are monitored periodically.

NB: *The maximum dosage of sodium valproate is 2.5 g daily in divided doses (prescribed as Epilim Chrono).*

Antipsychotics

(a) **Chlorpromazine:**
   1   Control of the psychotic components of psychotic depression.
   2   Usually brings the symptoms of acute mania under rapid control.

(b) Haloperidol:

Conventional antipsychotic drug of choice for mania – since it is less sedative and causes less postural hypotension, cf. chlorpromazine.

(c) Risperidone:

1 Licensed in the UK in 2004 for the treatment of mania in bipolar disorder:

    (i) Either as monotherapy or in combination with a mood stabiliser (lithium or valproate), no dose adjustment required.

    (ii) Co-administration with carbamazapine in bipolar mania not recommended.

    (iii) When initiating treatment, the starting dose is 2 mg o.d. on the first day, which may be increased to 3 mg o.d. on the second day in bipolar mania; due to high affinity for α_1-adrenergic receptors.

    (iv) Usual dose range 1 mg o.d. to 6 mg o.d., continued use must be evaluated and justified on an ongoing basis.

2 Some evidence it may be useful in the treatment of resistant depression – as an augmenting agent to SSRIs (by enhancing serotonin accumulation within the synapse), although there is no licence in this area.

(d) Olanzapine:

1 Licensed in the UK in 2003 as monotherapy for the treatment of acute mania (starting dose 15 mg daily) and also for the prophylaxis of bipolar affective disorder (starting dose 10 mg daily).

2 It may also be used in combination with a mood stabiliser for both the treatment of acute mania and the prophylaxis of bipolar affective disorder (starting dose 10 mg daily).

3 During treatment for acute mania and the prophylaxis of bipolar affective disorder, daily dosage may subsequently be adjusted on the basis of individual clinical status within the range 5–20 mg/day.

4 Some evidence it may be useful in the treatment of resistant depression – as an augmenting agent to SSRIs (by enhancing serotonergic accumulation within the synapse), although there is no licence in this area.

(e) Quetiapine:

1 Licensed in the UK in 2003 for the treatment of acute mania either as monotherapy or in combination with a mood stabiliser.

2 When initiating treatment in acute mania, the starting dose is 50 mg b.d., which is then increased over five days to 300 mg b.d. in adults; due to high affinity for α_1-adrenergic receptors. The maximum dose for acute mania is 400 mg b.d.

(f) Antipsychotic depot injections:

Prophylaxis of bipolar affective disorder in patients who have poor compliance with oral prophylactic medication (mood stabilisers) – depot medication certainly protects against hypomanic relapse and some clinicians believe it also protects against a subsequent depressive relapse; IM risperidone may be the 'depot' (long-acting intramuscular injection) of choice in patients with bipolar affective disorder who are poorly compliant with oral mood stabilisers.

NB: To prevent relapse of a depressive disorder (unipolar affective disorder), it is necessary to continue antidepressant medication for six months postclinical recovery after the first episode of the disorder, and for several (one to three) years postclinical recovery after two or more episodes of the disorder; to prevent relapse of mania (bipolar affective disorder), it is necessary to continue the mood stabilising medication for six to twelve months postclinical recovery after the first episode of the disorder, and for up to five years postclinical recovery after two or more episodes of the disorder; however, if the first episode of either a depressive disorder or mania is totally destructive to the patient's life, lifelong antidepressant or mood stabilising medication should be considered postclinical recovery as the patient cannot afford to have a relapse of their disorder.

Electroconvulsive therapy (ECT)

(a) The effects of ECT are best in severe depressive disorders, particularly those with marked biological and psychotic features of depression; the therapeutic agent is the convulsion.

(b) It is mainly the speed of action that distinguishes ECT from antidepressant drug treatment (the mood elevating effect with the latter takes two weeks to begin, cf. ECT where the mood elevating effect can begin within a few days); thus, ECT is particularly indicated in patients:
   (i)   who are actively suicidal
   (ii) who are not eating and drinking adequately
   (iii) who are very distressed by their symptoms.

(c) ECT may also be used in the acute treatment of refractory mania.

Psychosurgery

Psychosurgery is reserved for cases of chronic, refactory, incapacitating depression, unresponsive to other measures including ECT (at least two years of treatment with other measures should be tried including consideration for a second course of ECT).

Social – social manipulation

1 Rehousing.
2 Family support, e.g. nursery.

Psychological – depressive disorders

1 Psychotherapy:
  (a) Supportive psychotherapy:
      (i) Part of the management of every depressed patient.
      (ii) Intended to sustain patient until other treatments have their effects, or natural recovery occurs.
  (b) Individual dynamic psychotherapy:
      (i) Most clinicians restrict the use of individual dynamic psychotherapy to less severe cases. Occasionally those with severe depressive disorders which have been medically stabilised can be treated with individual dynamic psychotherapy.
      (ii) Intended to effect change in the patient by confrontation of defences; clarification; interpretations – new formulations of the problems.
  (c) Interpersonal psychotherapy – a systematic and standardised treatment approach to relationships and life problems.
  (d) Family therapy – aims to alleviate the problems that led to the disorder in the identified patient, rather than to achieve some ideal state of a healthy family.
2 Cognitive therapy:
  (a) As mentioned earlier, Beck suggests that a person who habitually adopts ways of thinking with depressed 'cognitive distortions' will be more likely to become depressed when faced with minor problems.
  (b) In cognitive therapy, the depressed 'cognitive distortions' are identified from present or recent experiences with the use of daily records (Beck's diaries).
  (c) The patient records such ideas and then learns to examine the evidence for and against them, i.e. tests out beliefs in real life.
  (d) The patient can be encouraged to undertake some of the pleasurable activities that were given up at the onset of depression.
  (e) In this way, the patient attempts 'cognitive restructuring', i.e. to identify, evaluate and change his/her distorted thoughts and associated behaviours.

Prognosis

I   Bipolar affective disorders:
1   In these disorders there has been at least one episode of mania, irrespective of whether or not there has been a depressive disorder.
2   Mean age of onset is about 30 years:
   (a)   But wide variation in age from late teens to late life.
   (b)   90% of cases begin before age of 50 (Angst, 1973).
3   Nearly all manic patients recover eventually.
4   Manic illnesses often recur, and subsequent depressive disorder is frequent.
5   The length of remission between episodes of illness becomes shorter up to the third attack, but does not change after that.
6   Personality is well-preserved between episodes of illness.

II   Unipolar affective disorders – nearly all young patients recover, though not all elderly patients do so.

CHAPTER 9
Schizophrenia

Classification

I   Hebephrenic schizophrenia:
1   Silly and childish behaviour.
2   Prominent affective symptoms and thought disorder.
3   Delusions common but unsystematised.
4   Hallucinations common but non-elaborate.
5   Occurs in adolescents and young adults.

II   Paranoid schizophrenia:
1   Prominent well-systematised persecutory or grandiose delusions and hallucinations.
2   Delusional jealousy.
3   Mood and thought processes relatively spared.
4   Patient may appear normal until his abnormal beliefs are uncovered.
5   More common with increasing age.

III Simple schizophrenia:
1   Insidious development of social withdrawal.
2   Odd behaviour and declining performance at work.
3   Absence of delusions, hallucinations and interference with thinking.

IV   Catatonic schizophrenia:
1   Stupor; excitement.
2   Waxy flexibility; catalepsy.
3   Echolalia; echopraxia.
4   Automatic obedience; stereotypy.
5   Ambitendence; mannerism.
6   Mitmachen; mitgehen.
7   Negativism; perseveration.

Epidemiology

I   Age – median age of onset:
1   Males – 28 years.
2   Females – 32 years.

II   **Sex** – equally common among men and women.
III   **Social class** – increased prevalence in lower social classes.
IV   **Season of birth** – increased incidence in winter births.
V   **Birth order** – increased incidence of low birth order if from large family.
VI   **Prevalence rate** – 1% in the general population.

Clinical features

I   The **acute syndrome (positive symptoms)** – main features:
  1 Delusions.
  2 Hallucinations.
  3 Interference with thinking.
  4 Incongruity of affect.
  5 Precipitated by too much social stimulation.
II   The **chronic syndrome (negative symptoms; defect state)** – main features:
  1 Apathy.
  2 Lack of drive and initiative, i.e. diminished volition.
  3 Social withdrawal.
  4 Deterioration of social behaviour, e.g. shouting obscenities in public.
  5 Slowness, i.e. underactivity.
  6 Poverty of speech.
  7 Poverty of thought.
  8 Schizophrenic or formal thought disorder (i.e. loosening of associations).
  9 Blunting of affect.
  10 Age disorientation.
  11 Precipitated by too little social stimulation.
  NB: Poverty of speech and blunting of affect are the core negative symptoms.
III **Schneider's first-rank symptoms of schizophrenia:**
  1 Particular forms of auditory hallucination:
    (a) Third person auditory hallucinations – two or more voices discussing or arguing about the subject with each other.
    (b) Running commentary – voices commenting on the subject's actions in the third person.
    (c) Thought echo (audible thoughts):
       (i)   Gedankenlautwerden – the patient experiences a voice speaking his own thoughts as he thinks them.
       (ii) Écho de la pensée – the patient experiences a voice repeating his own thoughts immediately after he has thought them.

2 Interference with thinking:
   (a) Thought insertion.
   (b) Thought withdrawal.
   (c) Thought broadcasting.
3 Other symptoms:
   (a) Primary delusion (delusional perception) – a false belief which arises fully formed as a sudden intuition, having no discernible connection with any previous interactions or experiences. Frequently preceded by a delusional mood, in which the patient feels something strange and threatening is happening, but is not sure exactly what.
   (b) Somatic hallucinations – hallucinatory sensations of sexual intercourse attributed to unwanted sexual interference by a persecutor or series of persecutors.
   (c) 'Made' volition.

IV Schneider's second-rank symptoms of schizophrenia:
   1 Secondary delusion – a false belief which arises from some preceding morbid experience, e.g. a prevailing mood, an existing delusion or a hallucination.
   2 Second person auditory hallucinations (abusive or derogatory) – the patient usually resents such comments; cf. depressive disorders, when the patient accepts them as justified.
   3 Visual, tactile, olfactory and gustatory hallucinations.
   4 Incongruity or blunting of affect.
   5 Formal thought disorder.
   6 Catatonic symptoms (disorders of motor activity) – *see* catatonic schizophrenia.

V Other clinical features of schizophrenia:
   1 Neologisms.
   2 Metonyms (paraphrasias) – the use of ordinary words in unusual ways.
   3 Abnormalities of mood – depression; euphoria; anxiety; irritability.
   4 Grandiose delusions.
   5 Persecutory delusions.
   6 Delusions of reference.
   7 Thought blocking.
   8 Concrete thinking – difficulty in dealing with abstract ideas.
   9 Lack of insight.

Aetiology

I **Genetic** – strong evidence for genetic aetiology provided by:
  1 Family studies – the prevalence rates of schizophrenia in relatives of a schizophrenic are as follows:

Relationship to schizophrenic	Prevalence rate
Parent of a schizophrenic	5%
Sibling of a schizophrenic	10%
Child of one schizophrenic parent	14%
Child of two schizophrenic parents	46%

  Cf. prevalence rate of 1% in the general population.

  2 Twin studies – concordance rate in MZ twins is 45%; cf. 10% in DZ twins (Gottesmann and Shields, 1972).
  3 Adoption studies – Heston (1966) studied 47 children whose mothers were schizophrenic, but who were adopted shortly after birth. These children were compared with similarly adopted children, whose mothers were non-schizophrenic – 14% of the group developed schizophrenia; cf. 0% of the controls.

II **Biochemical theories:**
  1 The dopamine theory of schizophrenia – schizophrenia results from overactivity of dopamine within the mesolimbic cortical bundle.
    (a) Evidence for:
      (i) Amphetamines increase dopamine release and can produce a paranoid psychosis similar to schizophrenia.
      (ii) Disulfiram inhibits dopamine-β-hydroxylase and can exacerbate schizophrenia.
      (iii) All effective neuroleptics block dopamine receptors; antipsychotic potency is related to the degree of antidopaminergic activity.
      (iv) Monoamine re-uptake inhibitors can exacerbate schizophrenia.
      (v) Post-mortem studies indicate increased dopamine levels in mesolimbic areas of schizophrenic brains.
    (b) Evidence against:
      (i) CSF studies fail to show increased metabolites of dopamine in schizophrenia; i.e. the levels of homovanillic acid (HVA) are reduced.
      (ii) Antipsychotics may raise HVA levels.
      (iii) Low-dose apomorphine, a dopamine stimulator, can lead to improvement in chronic schizophrenia.
      (iv) L-dopa can reduce the negative symptoms of schizophrenia.

2 The transmethylation theory of schizophrenia – abnormal methylated metabolites are formed in the brain due to aberrant methylation of monoamines, and produce the psychological symptoms of schizophrenia. This theory is based on the observation that mescaline, a hallucinogen, is an ortho-methylated derivative of dopamine.

   (a) Evidence for: the methyl donor methionine, when given in conjunction with an MAOI, exacerbates schizophrenic symptoms.

   (b) Evidence against: the supposed methyl acceptors nicotinamide and nicotinic acid are without therapeutic effect in the treatment of schizophrenia.

III **Psychological theories:**

1 Arousal – some schizophrenics are overaroused. This abnormality is more frequent among the more socially withdrawn chronic patients.

2 Attention and perception – schizophrenics cannot concentrate selectively on the important aspects of sensory input. An overwhelming input of stimuli may provide a basis for some of the perceptual abnormalities described by these patients.

3 Thought disorder:

   (a) Concrete thinking (Goldstein) – inability to think in abstract terms; concrete concepts are substituted.

   (b) Over-inclusiveness (Cameron) – inability to conserve conceptual boundaries, with the result that there is an incorporation of irrelevant ideas.

   (c) Personal construct theory (Kelly, Bannister) – schizophrenics have an abnormally loose personal construct system, which can be measured with the repertory grid. Abnormal constructs might have developed through repeated invalidations of the patient's previous attempts to make sense of the world, perhaps as a result of disordered family communication experienced in childhood.

4 Psychoanalytic theory:

   (a) Freud – schizophrenia is explained in terms of a withdrawal of libido from external objects. Since the withdrawal of libido makes the external world meaningless, the patient attempts to restore meaning by developing abnormal beliefs.

   (b) Klein – failure to pass through the 'paranoid–schizoid' position adequately is the basis for the later development of schizophrenia. In the 'paranoid–schizoid' position, the infant is thought to deal with innate aggressive impulses by splitting both his own ego and his representation of his mother into two incompatible parts, one wholly bad and the other wholly good. Only later does the child realise that the same person could be good at one time and bad at another.

(c)   Sullivan – schizophrenia is explained in terms of interpersonal difficulties.

5   Premorbid personality – schizophrenia is associated with schizoid personality traits in a minority of people (*see* Chapter 3).

IV   **Social processes:**

1   Farris and Dunham (1939) – found a raised incidence of schizophrenia in inner-city Chicago. This gave rise to the social causation hypothesis – poverty and deprivation in lower social class areas lead to schizophrenia.

2   Goldberg and Morrison (1963) – found that while schizophrenics were predominantly found in the lower social classes, they came from families which were distributed evenly throughout all social classes. This gave rise to the social drift hypothesis – schizophrenia results in the individual's slide down the social scale.

3   Odegaard (1932):
(a)   He showed an increased rate of hospital admissions for Norwegian immigrants in the United States, as compared to Norwegians at home, especially due to schizophrenia.
(b)   This stimulated debate between:
(i)   Social causation – environmental factors associated with migration lead to mental illness.
(ii)   Social selection – individuals prone to or suffering from mental illness tend to migrate.
(c)   Odegaard favoured social selection for schizophrenia.

4   Hare (1956) – schizophrenics often live alone, unmarried, with few friends, i.e. in social isolation.

5   Clausen and Kohn (1959) – such social isolation begins before the illness, sometimes in early childhood. Schizophrenics not isolated in early life were not isolated as adults.

V   **Abnormal family processes:**

I   Disordered family communications:
(a)   Bateson (1956) – features of a double bind:
(i)   Occurs when an instruction is given overtly, but contradicted by a second, more covert instruction, i.e. a parent conveys two conflicting and incompatible messages to their child at the same time.
(ii)   There is no escape from the situation is which the contradictory instructions are received.
(iii)   The double bind leaves the child able to make only ambiguous or meaningless responses.
(iv)   When this process persists, this was said to lead to schizophrenia.

    (b) Wynne and Singer (1963) – suggested that disrupted, non-sequential communications from and between parents lead to schizophrenia in their child.

2   Deviant role relationships:
    (a) Fromm–Reichmann (1948):
       (i)   He suggested the concept of the 'schizophrenogenic' mother, i.e. he found that the mothers of schizophrenics showed an excess of psychological abnormalities; cf. the mothers of neurotic patients and normal controls.
      (ii) He suggested that these abnormalities might be an important cause of the child's schizophrenia.
    (b) Lidz (1957) – two types of abnormal family pattern:
       (i)   Marital skew – in which one parent yielded to the other's (usually the mother's) eccentricities, which dominated the family.
      (ii) Marital schism – in which the parents maintained contrary views so that the child has divided loyalties. The inconsistencies, contradictions and lack of role models were said to lead to schizophrenia.

3   High expressed emotion (Vaughn and Leff, 1976):
    (a) Refers to relatives in the patient's family making critical comments, expressing hostility, or showing signs of emotional over-involvement.
    (b) The relapse rate is highest in patients who are exposed to high expressed emotion ('EE'), have more than 35 hours per week face-to-face contact with the key (high 'EE') relative, and are not complying with their antipsychotic medication.

VI **Neurological abnormalities:**
1   Non-localising ('soft') neurological signs:
    (a) Astereognosis.
    (b) Dysgraphaesthesia.
    (c) Gait abnormalities.
    (d) Clumsiness.
    These abnormalities reflect defects in the integration of proprioceptive and other sensory information.

2   Thickening of the corpus callosum – some suggestion of impairment of interhemispheric transfer in schizophrenics.

3   Ventricular enlargement:
    (a) Widening of sulci, atrophy of cerebellar vermis.
    (b) Some evidence that patients with ventricular enlargement have more negative symptoms of schizophrenia.
    (c) Some evidence that such patients perform poorly on tests of intellectual function.

4 Changes in the EEG:
  (a) Increased theta activity.
  (b) Fast activity.
  (c) Paroxysmal activity.
5 Virus-like material – isolated from the CSF of schizophrenics. Virus infection may be a major cause of schizophrenia.
VII **Life event studies** – schizophrenics experience more life events over normal controls in the three weeks prior to the onset of acute symptoms of schizophrenia (Brown and Birley,1968).
VIII **Body build (Kretschmer)** – patients of asthenic (lean and narrow) build are particularly prone to schizophrenia.

Diagnosis

I Definite evidence of Schneiderian first-rank symptoms – indicates a diagnosis of schizophrenia, provided that there is no evidence of an organic disorder.
II In the absence of Schneiderian first-rank symptoms – a diagnosis of schizophrenia can still be made if there is evidence of a prolonged course together with definite evidence of the negative symptoms of schizophrenia.
III In the absence of Schneiderian first-rank symptoms – a diagnosis of schizophrenia can still be considered if the nature of the delusional beliefs is very bizarre.

Differential diagnosis

I **Exclude organic disorders:**
  1 Among younger patients:
    (a) Drug-induced psychosis:
      (i) Amphetamine abuse.
      (ii) Alcohol abuse.
    (b) Temporal lobe epilepsy (complex partial seizures).
  2 Among older patients:
    (a) Acute organic syndrome – e.g. encephalitis.
    (b) Dementia.
    (c) Diffuse brain diseases – e.g. general paralysis of the insane (GPI).
  3 In addition – a schizophrenic syndrome can occur post-partum and in the post-operative period.

II   Exclude affective disorders.
III Exclude personality disorders.

Management

Physical

A CONVENTIONAL ANTIPSYCHOTICS

I   CHLORPROMAZINE
  (a) **Mode of action**
    1   Dopamine antagonist; blocks D_2-receptors in the mesolimbic cortical bundle – which mediates the antipsychotic action of chlorpromazine.
    2   It also has several other biochemical actions, which mediate the side-effects of chlorpromazine:
      (i)   Dopamine blocking activity at other sites (*see* later).
      (ii) Antiserotonergic activity.
      (iii) α_1-adrenergic receptor antagonist.
      (iv) Muscarinic M_1-receptor antagonist.
      (v)   Histamine H_1-receptor antagonist.
  (b) **Indications**
    1   Control and maintenance therapy in schizophrenia (usual maintenance dose 50 mg b.d. to 100 mg t.d.s.; maximum dose 1 g daily in divided doses).
    2   Chlorpromazine is more sedative and causes less extra pyramidal side-effects, cf. haloperidol – thus, chlorpromazine was the drug of choice for schizophrenia (before the advent of atypical antipsychotics).
  (c) **Adverse effects**
    1   Extra pyramidal side-effects (EPSEs) – mediated by dopamine-blocking activity at D_2-receptors in the nigrostriatal pathway:
      (i)   Acute dystonic reactions.
      (ii) Akathesia.
      (iii) Pseudoparkinsonism.
      (iv) Tardive dyskinesia.
    2   Hyperprolactinaemia – mediated by dopamine blocking activity at D_2-receptors in the tubero-infundibular system – galactorrhoea in both women and men.
    3   Antiserotonergic side-effect: depression.

4 Antiadrenergic side-effects (due to blockade of α_1-adrenergic receptors):
   (i)   Postural hypotension.
   (ii)   Failure of ejaculation.
   (iii) Sedation.
5 Anticholinergic side-effects (due to blockade of muscarinic M_1-receptors):
   (i)   Dry mouth.
   (ii)   Blurred vision.
   (iii) Constipation.
   (iv)   Urinary retention.
   (v)   Tachycardia.
   (vi)   Impotence.
   (vii) Exacerbation of glaucoma.
6 Antihistaminergic side-effect (due to blockade of histamine H_1-receptors): sedation.
   NB: Sedation is mainly mediated through anti-adrenergic activity.
7 Impaired temperature regulation:
   (i)   Hypothermia.
   (ii)   Hyperpyrexia.
8 Neuroleptic malignant syndrome (NMS).
9 Bone marrow suppression – leucopenia.
10 Skin photosensitivity and pigmentation.
11 Cardiac arrhythmias.
12 Cholestatic jaundice.
13 Seizures (due to lowering of the convulsive threshold).
14 Weight gain.

II **HALOPERIDOL**
   (a) **Mode of action**
      1 Greater dopamine blocking activity.
      2 Less antiadrenergic activity.   cf. chlorpromazine
      3 Less anticholinergic activity.
   (b) **Adverse effects**
      1 More EPSE.
      2 Less sedation.
      3 Less postural hypotension.   cf. chlorpromazine
      4 Fewer anticholinergic side-effects.
      5 NMS.
      6 Danger of severe EPSE with haloperidol if a daily dose in excess of 20 mg is combined with lithium carbonate at a serum level of greater than 0.8 mmol/l.
      7 ECG changes at high dose – torsade de pointes.

8   Recently the maximum BNF recommended dose of haloperidol has been heavily reduced to:
(i)   30 mg daily in divided doses if taken orally.
(ii)   18 mg daily in divided doses as an intramuscular injection.
This is due to EPSE at higher doses.

III TRIFLUOPERAZINE

(a) Mode of action
1   Greater dopamine blocking activity. ⎫
2   Less antiadrenergic activity.   ⎬   cf. chlorpromazine
3   Less anticholinergic activity.   ⎭

(b) Indications
1   Useful in psychotic patients where sedation is undesirable (i.e. retarded psychotic patients) since it is less sedative – cf. chlorpromazine.
2   Useful in psychotic patients with intractable auditory hallucinations; usual dose range 5 mg b.d. to 5 mg t.d.s.

(c) Adverse effects
1   More EPSE.   ⎫
2   Less sedation.   ⎪
3   Less postural hypotension.   ⎬   cf. chlorpromazine
4   Less anticholinergic side-effects. ⎭

IV SULPIRIDE

(a) Mode of action
1   Low doses – thought to block presynaptic dopamine D_3- and D_4-autoreceptors.
2   High doses – blocks postsynaptic dopamine receptors; more specific blocker of D_2-receptors, cf. D_1-receptors.

(b) Indications
1   Low doses – may have an alerting effect on schizophrenic patients with negative symptoms such as apathy and social withdrawal (optimum dosage 400 mg b.d.).
2   High doses – useful in schizophrenic patients with florid positive symptoms such as delusions and hallucinations (optimum dosage 800 mg b.d.).

(c) Adverse effects
1   Less EPSE – cf. chlorpromazine.
2   Less sedation – cf. chlorpromazine.
3   Tendency to cause galactorrhoea.

B ATYPICAL ANTIPSYCHOTICS

I   **RISPERIDONE**
Introduced into the UK in 1993.

(a) **Mode of action**
1   Potent dopamine D_2-receptor antagonist; in addition it has a regional preference for blocking D_2 receptors in the mesolimbic cortical bundle, cf. the nigrostriatal pathway.
2   Potent serotonin $5HT_{2A}$-receptor antagonist.
3   Low affinity for serotonin $5HT_{2C}$-receptors.
4   Potent α_1-adrenergic receptor antagonist.
5   No appreciable affinity for muscarinic M_1-receptors.
6   Low affinity for histamine H_1-receptors.

(b) **Indications**
1   Treatment of both the positive and negative symptoms of schizophrenia; it appears efficacious in treating both sets of symptoms equally well (usual dose range 4 mg o.d. to 6 mg o.d for maintenance treatment in adults).
Treatment of negative symptoms is mediated by blockade of serotonin $5HT_{2A}$-receptors.
2   Alleviation of affective symptoms associated with schizophrenia – mediated by blockade of serotonin $5HT_{2A}$-receptors.
3   Useful in maintenance treatment of schizophrenic patients who dislike antipsychotic depot injections – it has recently been given a licence such that it need only be taken once a day to prevent relapse of schizophrenia.
NB: Risperidone is available in the UK as an oral preparation (including a quicklet which may be placed on the tongue or allowed to dissolve or dissolved in water); however IM risperidone, a long-acting intramuscular injection form of risperidone, was launched in the UK in 2002 (see later under antipsychotic depot injections).

(c) **Adverse effects**
1   Less EPSE (at doses up to and including 6 mg o.d.), cf. other antipsychotic drugs; this benefit may be lost at doses of and over 8 mg o.d. – above this dose, it requires twice-daily dosing, i.e. the next increment is 5 mg b.d. and this may be gradually increased up to a maximum of 8 mg b.d.
2   Dose dependent elevation in prolactin levels, although these are not necessarily related to the possible sexual side-effects.
3   Minimal weight again due to low affinity for serotonin $5HT_{2C}$-receptors.

4 Postural hypotension – therefore when initiating treatment, the starting dose is 2 mg o.d. on the first day, which may be increased to 4 mg o.d. on the second day in schizophrenia (slower titration over a week appropriate in some patients); due to high affinity for α_1-adrenergic receptors.

5 No appreciable anticholinergic side-effects.

6 Side-effects include agitation and insomnia due to possible low affinity for histamine H_1-receptors.

7 Some ECG changes (prolongation of the QT interval). However, there is no requirement for routine ECG monitoring.

8 Not associated with agranulocytosis.

9 Gastrointestinal side-effects – nausea, dyspepsia, abdominal pain.

10 More akathesia, cf. chlorpromazine.

II OLANZAPINE

Introduced into the UK in 1996.

(a) Mode of action

1 Potent dopamine D_2-receptor antagonist; it preferentially blocks D_2 receptors in the mesolimbic cortical bundle, cf. the nigrostriatal pathway.

2 Potent serotonin $5HT_{2A}$-receptor antagonist.

3 High affinity for serotonin $5HT_{2C}$-receptors.

4 Moderate affinity for α_1-adrenergic receptors.

5 High affinity for muscarinic M_1-receptors.

6 High affinity for histamine H_1-receptors.

(b) Indications

1 Treatment of both the positive and negative symptoms of schizophrenia, and affective symptoms associated with schizophrenia (starting dose 10 mg daily; dose range 5–20 mg daily for maintenance treatment).

2 Maintenance treatment of schizophrenia (once-per-day dosing).

NB: Olanzapine is available in the UK as an oral preparation (including a velotab which may be placed on the tongue and allowed to dissolve or dissolved in water); however, IM olanzapine, for use in rapid tranquillisation was launched in the UK in 2004 (see later under the acutely disturbed patient in Chapter 13).

(c) Adverse effects

1 EPSE usually mild and transient if present – responds to dose reduction or to an antimuscarinic drug.

2 Sometimes associated with elevation in prolactin level. However, associated clinical manifestations are rare, cf. risperidone.

3 Significant weight gain due to high affinity for serotonin $5HT_{2C}$-receptors; treatment-emergent diabetes mellitus does not appear to be associated with weight gain.

4   Some postural hypotension. However, treatment can be initiated at a therapeutic dose (10 mg daily) without the need to build up from a starting dose due to moderate affinity for α_1-adrenergic receptors.

5   Anticholinergic side-effects: dry mouth may occur.

6   Side-effects include sedation due to high affinity for histamine H_1-receptors.

7   Not generally associated with clinically significant prolongation of the QT interval. No requirement for routine ECG monitoring.

8   Not associated with agranulocytosis.

9   Transient, asymptomatic elevation of hepatic transaminases has been seen in association with olanzapine therapy. However, there is no CSM recommendation to routinely monitor LFTs (liver function tests).

III   QUETIAPINE

Introduced into the UK in 1997.

(a) **Mode of action**

1   Weak affinity for dopamine D_2-receptors – similar to clozapine.

2   Low affinity for serotonin $5HT_{2A}$-receptors.

3   Very low affinity for serotonin $5HT_{2C}$-receptors.

4   High affinity for α_1-adrenergic receptors.

5   No appreciable affinity for muscarinic M_1-receptors.

6   High affinity for histamine H_1-receptors.

(b) **Indications**

1   Treatment of the symptoms of schizophrenia (positive, negative and affective).

2   Maintenance treatment of schizophrenia (twice-per-day dosing; usual dose range 150 mg b.d. to 225 mg b.d. for maintenance treatment).

3   May be effective in the treatment of resistant schizophrenia at higher doses (250 mg b.d. to 375 mg b.d.), i.e. in patients who have failed to respond to another atypical antipsychotic (risperidone, olanzapine).

NB: Quetiapine is only currently available in the UK as an oral preparation.

(c) **Adverse effects**

1   EPSE comparable with placebo across the dose range (up to, and including, the maximum dose of 375 mg b.d.).

2   Prolactin level comparable with placebo across the dose range (up to, and including, the maximum dose).

3   Minimal weight gain due to very low affinity for serotonin $5HT_{2C}$-receptors.

4   Postural hypotension – therefore when initiating treatment in schizophrenia, the starting dose is 25 mg b.d., which is then increased over four days to 150 mg b.d. in adults; due to high affinity for α_1-adrenergic receptors.

5   No appreciable anticholinergic side-effects.

6   Side-effects include headaches and somnolence; latter due to high affinity for histamine H_1-receptors.

7   Some ECG changes (prolongation of the QT interval). However, there is no requirement for routine ECG monitoring.

8   Not associated with agranulocytosis.

9   Some disturbance in LFTs. However, there is no requirement for the routine monitoring of LFTs.

10 Requires twice-daily dosing, cf. risperidone (up to 8 mg daily), olanzapine and aripiprazole which require once-daily dosing; this may reduce compliance in patients taking quetiapine for the long-term treatment of schizophrenia.

IV AMISULPRIDE
Introduced in the UK in 1997.

(a) **Mode of action**

1   Blocks dopamine D_3-receptors (mainly presynaptic) and dopamine D_2-receptors (mainly postsynaptic); limbic selective.

2   No affinity for serotonin $5HT_{2A}$-receptors.

3   No affinity for serotonin $5HT_{2C}$-receptors.

4   No affinity for α_1-adrenergic receptors.

5   No affinity for muscarinic M_1-receptors.

6   No affinity for histamine H_1-receptors.

(b) **Indications**

1   Treatment of schizophrenic patients with florid positive symptoms or a mixture of positive and negative symptoms (usual dose range 200 mg b.d. to 400 mg b.d.; maximum dosage 600 mg b.d.); it can be initiated at 400 mg b.d. for florid positive symptoms.

2   Treatment of schizophrenic patients with predominantly negative symptoms (dose range 50 mg to 300 mg daily with an optimum dosage of 100 mg once a day).

NB: Amisulpride is currently only available in the UK as an oral preparation.

(c) **Adverse effects**

1   Lower potential for causing EPSE, cf. conventional antipsychotics; however, this benefit is lost at the maximum dosage.

2   Reversible elevation in prolactin level associated with clinical manifestations; not dose dependent and comparable to conventional antipsychotics.

3   Low weight gain due to lack of affinity for serotonin $5HT_{2C}$-receptors.

4   Some postural hypotension. However, treatment can be initiated at a therapeutic dose (200 mg b.d. for positive symptoms with or without negative symptoms) without the need to build up from a starting dose; due to lack of affinity for α_1-adrenergic receptors.

5   No appreciable anticholinergic side-effects.

6   Side-effects include insomnia, anxiety and agitation.

7   Some ECG changes. However, there is no requirement for routine ECG monitoring.

8   Not associated with agranulocytosis.

9   There is no requirement for the routine monitoring of LFTs.

10 May be the atypical antipsychotic of choice in patients with diabetes mellitus – due to its lack of affinity for serotonin $5HT_{2C}$-receptors.

11 Requires twice-daily dosing, cf. risperidone (up to 8 mg daily), olanzapine and aripiprazole which require once-daily dosing; this may reduce compliance in patients taking amisulpiride for the long-term treatment of schizophrenia.

V   **ARIPIPRAZOLE**

Introduced into the UK in 2004.

(a) **Mode of action**

1   Partial agonist at dopamine D_2-receptors:
   (i)   Acts as a dopamine D_2-receptor agonist on presynaptic autoreceptors.
   (ii) Acts as a dopamine D_2-receptor antagonist on postsynaptic receptors.
   (iii) Aripiprazole acts as a dopamine system stabiliser in both hypodopaminergic and hyperdopaminergic conditions. As shown in animal models *in vivo*, stabilisation of the dopamine system is proposed to provide antipsychotic efficacy with minimal adverse effects.

2   Partial agonist at serotonin $5HT_{1A}$-receptors:
   (i)   May protect against dopamine-mediated adverse effects.
   (ii) May provide anxiolytic activity.

3   High affinity for serotonin $5HT_{2A}$-receptors.

4   Low affinity for serotonin $5HT_{2C}$-receptors.

5   Low affinity for α_1-adrenergic receptors.

6   Low affinity for muscarinic M_1-receptors.

7   Low affinity for histamine H_1-receptors.

(b) **Indications**

1   Treatment of the positive symptoms of schizophrenia – due to its action as a dopamine D_2-receptor antagonist in the mesolimbic area (where dopamine is excessive).

2   Treatment of the negative symptoms of schizophrenia – due to its action as a dopamine D_2-receptor agonist in the mesocortical area (where dopamine is deficient).

NB: The dosing is 15–30 mg mane; aripiprazole is currently only available in the UK as an oral preparation.

(c)   **Adverse effects**

1   EPSE comparable with placebo.

2   Prolactin level comparable with placebo.

3   Minimum weight gain due to low affinity for serotonin $5HT_{2C}$-receptors.

4   Some postural hypotension. However, treatment can be initiated at a therapeutic dose (15 mg) without the need to build up from a starting dose; due to low affinity for α_1-adrenergic receptors.

5   No appreciable anticholinergic side-effects.

6   Side-effects include insomnia, nausea, akathisia and the risk of seizures.

7   Not associated with ECG changes – therefore no requirement for routine ECG monitoring.

8   Not associated with agranulocytosis.

9   No requirement for the routine monitoring of LFTs.

10   No dose adjustments required in those with renal or hepatic impairment.

VI   **ZOTEPINE**

Introduced into the UK in 1998.

(a)   **Mode of action**

1   Moderate affinity for dopamine D_2-receptors.

2   High affinity for serotonin $5HT_{2A}$-receptors.

3   High affinity for serotonin $5HT_{2C}$-receptors.

4   Low affinity for α_1-adrenergic receptors.

5   Potent noradrenaline re-uptake inhibitor.

6   Low affinity for muscarinic M_1-receptors.

7   High affinity for histamine H_1-receptors.

(b)   **Indications**

1   Treatment of the symptoms of schizophrenia – it has a general licence for this, i.e. it is not specifically licensed for any individual set of symptoms (positive, negative or affective). However, it may have antidepressant effects due to its action as a potent noradrenaline re-uptake inhibitor.

2   It is initiated in adults at the therapeutic dose of 25 mg t.d.s.; if further clinical improvement is required this may be increased to 50 mg t.d.s.; it may be further increased to a maximum of 100 mg t.d.s. if required.

NB: Zotepine is currently only available in the UK as an oral preparation.

(c) **Adverse effects**

1 May have lower potential for causing EPSE, cf. conventional antipsychotics.

2 Sometimes associated with elevation in prolactin levels. However, associated clinical manifestations are rare.

3 Significant weight gain due to high affinity for serotonin $5HT_{2C}$-receptors.

4 Some postural hypotension. However, treatment can be initiated at a therapeutic dose without the need to build up from a starting dose; due to low affinity for α_1-adrenergic receptors.

5 Dry mouth due to potent noradrenaline re-uptake inhibition.

6 Side-effects include sedation due to high affinity for histamine H_1-receptors.

7 Other side-effects include asthenia, constipation, tachycardia, significant weight gain and seizures.

8 ECG changes (prolongation of the QT interval) associated with a possible increased risk of toxicity. In view of this, CSM recommends an ECG prior to commencing treatment in patients at risk of arrhythmias. Zotepine should therefore be used with caution in patients with clinically significant cardiac disease.

9 Sometimes associated with neutropenia. Therefore if an infection occurs, a full blood count should be checked.

10 Sometimes associated with elevation in hepatic transaminases. Therefore in patients with known hepatic impairment, liver function tests should be monitored weekly for the first three months.

11 Zotepine is uricosuric, therefore it should not be started within three weeks of resolution of an episode of acute gout.

12 Requires dosing three times a day, cf. risperidone (up to 8 mg daily), olanzapine and aripiprazole which require once-daily dosing; this may reduce compliance in patients taking zotepine for the long-term treatment of schizophrenia.

VII CLOZAPINE

(a) **Mode of action**

1 Moderate affinity for dopamine D_2-receptors.

2 More active at dopamine D_4-receptors, cf. other antipsychotics.

3 High affinity for serotonin $5HT_{2A}$-receptors.

4 High affinity for serotonin $5HT_{2C}$-receptors.

5 High affinity for α_1-adrenergic receptors.

6 High affinity for muscarinic M_1-receptors.

7 High affinity for muscarinic M_4-receptors.

8 High affinity for histamine H_1-receptors.

(b) **Indications**

The treatment of schizophrenia in patients unresponsive to, or intolerant of, conventional antipsychotic drugs; at least one drug from two chemically distinct classes should be given a full therapeutic trial before considering clozapine (the atypical antipsychotics may be used as first line treatment of schizophrenia); in addition, it may be worth considering a course of electroconvulsive therapy (ECT) before starting clozapine therapy, since this can be an effective treatment in resistant schizophrenia (particularly when a significant affective component is present).

NB:

(i) *Clozapine treatment must only be instituted by psychiatrists registered with the Clozaril Patient Monitoring Service (CPMS).*

(ii) *Clozapine is currently only available in the UK as an oral preparation.*

(c) **Adverse effects**

1 Less EPSE, cf. conventional antipsychotics.

2 Asymptomatic rise in serum prolactin.

3 Significant weight gain due to high affinity for serotonin $5HT_{2C}$-receptors; treatment-emergent diabetes mellitus does not appear to be associated with weight gain.

4 Postural hypotension with risk of collapse – therefore treatment should be initiated with a starting dose and then gradually increased over 14–21 days to 300 mg daily in divided doses; usual dose 200–450 mg daily (max. 900 mg daily).

5 More anticholinergic side-effects: hypersalivation due to high affinity for muscarinic M_4-receptors in the salivary glands is common; other atropinic side-effects due to muscarinic M_1-receptor blockade also occur.

6 Side-effects include sedation due to high affinity for histamine H_1-receptors.

7 Other side-effects include fits and rare instances of myocarditis.

8 Some ECG changes. However, there is no requirement for routine ECG monitoring.

9 It causes agranulocytosis (life-threatening) in 2–3% of patients taking the drug – its use is therefore restricted to patients registered with the Clozaril Patient Monitoring Service (CPMS) whereby the patient has regular full blood counts to detect any possible agranulocytosis; should this occur, the clozapine must be stopped.

10 No requirement for the routine monitoring of LFTs.

11 Requires twice-daily dosing, cf. risperidone (up to 8 mg daily), olanzapine and aripiprazole which require once-daily dosing; this may reduce compliance in patients taking clozapine for the

long-term treatment of schizophrenia (as may the requirement for regular full blood counts).

C ANTIPSYCHOTIC DEPOT INJECTIONS

IN GENERAL
  (a) **Mode of action**
       Long-acting depot injections administered intramuscularly as an oily injection and slowly released into the bloodstream.
  (b) **Indication**
       For maintenance therapy of schizophrenia – more conveniently given than oral antipsychotic preparations ensuring better patient compliance.
  (c) **Adverse effects**
       1   Initially patients should always be given a test dose injection to ensure that the patient does not experience undue side-effects or any idiosyncratic reactions to the medication or formulation.
       2   They may give rise to a higher incidence of EPSE – cf. oral antipsychotic preparations.

MORE SPECIFICALLY
1   **FLUPHENAZINE DECANOATE**
  (a) **Indications**
       Useful in treating agitated or aggressive schizophrenic patients.
  (b) **Adverse effects**
       Contraindicated in severely depressed states – in view of its tendency to cause depression.
2   **FLUPENTHIXOL DECANOATE**
  (a) **Indications**
       Useful in treating retarded or withdrawn schizophrenic patients – in view of its apparent alerting nature.
  (b) **Adverse effects**
       Not suitable for the treatment of agitated or aggressive schizophrenic patients – since it can cause over-excitement in such patients in view of its alerting nature.
3   **ZUCLOPENTHIXOL DECANOATE**
  (a) **Indications**
       Useful in treating agitated or aggressive schizophrenic patients.
  (b) **Adverse effects**
       Not suitable for the treatment of retarded or withdrawn schizophrenic patients – since it may exacerbate psychomotor retardation in such patients in view of its sedative nature.

4 **HALOPERIDOL DECANOATE**
   (a) **Indications**
   Maintenance treatment in schizophrenia; usually four-weekly administration.

5 **PIPOTHIAZINE PALMITATE**
   (a) **Indications**
   Maintenance treatment in schizophrenia; four-weekly administration.
   (b) **Adverse effects**
   Allegedly lower EPSE, cf. other conventional antipsychotic depot injections.

6 **IM RISPERIDONE**
   (a) **Indications**
   1 The world's first ever atypical antipsychotic long-acting intramuscular injection – launched in the UK in 2002.
   2 Licensed for the treatment of both the positive and the negative symptoms of schizophrenia; it also alleviates affective symptoms associated with schizophrenia; two-weekly administration.
   (b) **Adverse effects**
   Less ESPE, cf. other conventional antipsychotic depot injections.

ELECTROCONVULSIVE THERAPY (ECT)

I The traditional indications for ECT in the treatment of schizophrenia are:
   (a) The stupor or excitement of catatonic schizophrenia.
   (b) Severe depressive symptoms accompanying schizophrenia.
II ECT can also an effective treatment in resistant schizophrenia (particularly when a significant affective component is present); thus, it may be worth considering a course of ECT before starting clozapine therapy in the treatment of resistant schizophrenia.

Social

1 Work with relatives – counselling should be beneficial to families, especially when directed at reducing their expressed emotion; the patient may need to be separated from this.
2 Rehabilitation of the patient – using: day hospitals; half-way houses; sheltered workshops. Understimulation or overstimulation of the patient should be avoided.

Psychological

1   Supportive psychotherapy – supportive psychotherapy, counselling and advice to the patient are always required.
2   Social skills training:
  (a) Technique:
    (i) Social skills training aims to modify a patient's social behaviour in order to help overcome difficulties in forming and/or maintaining relationships with other people; in addition to improving social competence, it may also improve the subject's overall psychological adjustment.
    (ii) The procedure is applied to patients with social deficits consequent upon schizophrenia.
    (iii) Video recordings can be used to define and rate elements of the patient's behaviour in standard social encounters.
    (iv) The patient is then taught more appropriate behaviour by a combination of direct instruction, modelling, video-feedback and role reversal.
  (b) Indication: patients with chronic schizophrenia as part of a rehabilitation programme.
3   Token economy (positive reinforcement):
  (a) Technique:
    (i) This system uses positive and negative reinforcement to alter behaviour.
    (ii) Behaviours necessary for effective independent living are specified.
    (iii) A unit of exchange (the token) is specific and its presentation to patient is made contingent upon the occurrence of the required behaviour, i.e. if the patient produces the required behaviour, he receives a number of tokens (positive reinforcement); if the patient fails to produce the required behaviour, the tokens are withheld (negative reinforcement).
    (iv) It is usual to give tokens that can be used to purchase goods or privileges.
  (b) Indication: patients with chronic schizophrenia as part of a rehabilitation programme.
4   Cognitive therapy – can help to:
  (a) Alleviate residual psychotic symptoms, e.g. hallucinations.
  (b) Improve insight.
NB: Cognitive therapy should be used in conjunction with antipsychotic medication.

Prognosis

I   'The rule of quarters':
    1   25% – remit completely after a first attack of schizophrenia with no further symptoms.
    2   25% – show good social recovery but with some persistence of symptoms.
    3   25% – show partial social recovery with persistence of symptoms.
    4   25% – follow a steadily downhill course with social deterioration, personality deterioration and, in some cases, ending with the defect state.

II   Good prognostic features:
    1 Acute onset.
    2 Presence of a precipitating factor.
    3 Prominence of affective symptoms.
    4 Older age at onset.
    5 Short episode.
    6 No past psychiatric history.
    7 Good premorbid personality.
    8 Good psychosexual adjustment.
    9 Good social relationships.
    10 Good work record.
    11 Married.

III   Causes of relapse:
    1 Iatrogenic relapse, i.e. the doctor reducing the patient's medication in an attempt to minimise the risk of tardive dyskinesia – commonest cause of relapse.
    2 Non-compliance with medication – second commonest cause of relapse.
    3 High 'EE' – third commonest cause of relapse.

CHAPTER 10

Organic disorders

Classification

I   Acute organic disorder (delirium):
   1   Acute onset.
   2   Fluctuating course.
II Chronic organic disorder (dementia):
   1   Insidious onset.
   2   Steady progressive course.

Clinical features

I   Acute organic disorder:
   1   Consciousness – impairment of consciousness recognised by:
     (a)   Slowness.
     (b)   Uncertainty about the time of day.
     (c)   Poor concentration.
   2   Behaviour – two possible forms:
     (a)   Overactivity, noisiness, repetitive purposeless movements.
     (b)   Inactivity, slowness, repetitive purposeless movements.
   3   Speech – reduced speech.
   4   Mood:
     (a)   Anxiety.
     (b)   Irritability.
     (c)   Depression.
     (d)   Lability of mood.
     (e)   Perplexed or frightened and agitated.
   5   Thought:
     (a)   Slow and muddled – but often rich in content.
     (b)   Ideas of reference and persecutory delusions – transient and poorly elaborated.
     (c)   Perseveration.

6 Perception:
(a) Visual illusions, visual misinterpretations and visual hallucinations – may have a fantastic content.
(b) Tactile and auditory hallucinations.
(c) Depersonalisation and derealisation.
7 Cognition:
(a) Disorientation in time and place.
(b) Disturbance of memory – affecting registration, retention, recall and new learning.
8 Insight – impaired.

II **Chronic organic disorder:**
1 Consciousness – no impairment of consciousness (i.e. clear consciousness). Global impairment of cerebral functions – i.e. generalised impairment of intellect, personality and memory.
2 Behaviour:
(a) Shrinkage of the milieu – reduction of interests.
(b) Organic orderliness – rigid and stereotyped routines.
(c) Catastrophic reaction – when the person is taxed beyond restricted abilities, there is a sudden explosion of anger or other emotion.
3 Speech:
(a) Syntactical errors and nominal dysphasia.
(b) Eventually patient may utter only meaningless noises or become mute.
4 Mood:
(a) Anxiety.
(b) Irritability.
(c) Depression.
(d) Lability of mood.
5 Thought:
(a) Slow and impoverished in content.
(b) Persecutory delusions.
(c) Perseveration.
(d) Concrete thinking.
6 Perception – hallucinations.
7 Cognition:
(a) Disorientation in time, place and person.
(b) Impaired attention and concentration.
(c) Disturbance of memory:
(i) Forgetfulness.
(ii) Difficulty in new learning is generally the most conspicuous sign.

       (iii) Memory loss is more obvious for recent than for remote events.

       (iv) Patients may use confabulation to hide memory deficits, i.e. apparent recollection of imaginary events and experiences.

8 Insight – impaired.

Aetiology

I   Acute organic disorder:

  1 Alcohol/drugs:
     (a) Alcohol or other drug intoxication (e.g. L-dopa, anticholinergics, anxiolytic–hypnotics, anticonvulsants, opiates).
     (b) Withdrawal of alcohol or other drugs.

  2 Metabolic causes:
     (a) Uraemia.
     (b) Electrolyte imbalance (e.g. hypercalcaemia).
     (c) Cardiac failure.
     (d) Respiratory failure.
     (e) Hepatic failure.
     (f) Acute intermittent porphyria.
     (g) Systemic lupus erythematosus (SLE).

  3 Endocrine causes:
     (a) Hyperthyroidism.
     (b) Hypothyroidism.
     (c) Hypoparathyroidism.
     (d) Hypopituitarism.
     (e) Hypoglycaemia.

  4 Infective causes:
     (a) Intercranial infection:
       (i) Encephalitis.
       (ii) Meningitis.
     (b) Systemic infection:
       (i) Septicaemia.
       (ii) Pneumonia.

  5 Other intracranial causes:
     (a) Space-occupying lesion.
     (b) Raised intracranial pressure.

  6 Vitamin deficiency:
     (a) B_1 (thiamine) – Wernicke's encephalopathy.
     (b) B_{12}.
     (c) Nicotinic acid.

7 Head injury.
8 Heavy metals – heavy metal intoxication (e.g. lead, manganese).
9 Epilepsy.

II **Chronic organic disorder:**
  1 Degenerative causes:
    (a) Senile dementia of the Alzheimer type (SDAT).
    (b) Alzheimer's disease.
    (c) Multi-infarct dementia (MID).
    (d) Pick's disease.
    (e) Parkinson's disease.
    (f) Huntington's chorea.
    (g) Normal pressure hydrocephalus (communicating hydrocephalus).
    (h) Multiple sclerosis (disseminated sclerosis).
    (i) Creutzfeldt–Jakob's disease (CJD).
    (j) Subacute spongiform encephalopathy.
    (k) Subcortical dementia.
    (l) Punch drunk syndrome.
  2 Metabolic causes:
    (a) Sustained uraemia.
    (b) Electrolyte imbalance (e.g. hypocalcaemia).
    (c) Chronic respiratory failure.
    (d) Chronic hepatic failure.
    (e) Chronic renal failure.
    (f) Wilson's disease.
    (g) SLE.
  3 Endocrine causes – hypothyroidism.
  4 Infective causes – intracranial infection:
    (a) Encephalitis.
    (b) Neurosyphilis – general paralysis of the insane (GPI).
    (c) Cerebral sarcoidosis.
  5 Other intracranial causes – space-occupying lesion (e.g. tumour, subdural haematoma).
  6 Vitamin deficiency – sustained lack of:
    (a) B_{12} – subacute combined degeneration of the cord.
    (b) Nicotinic acid – pellagra.
  7 Head injury.
  8 Alcohol/heavy metals – alcohol or heavy metal intoxication (e.g. lead, arsenic, thallium).
  9 Anoxia:
    (a) Cardiac arrest.
    (b) Carbon monoxide poisoning.
    (c) Anaemia.
    (d) Post-anaesthesia.

Diagnosis

I Senile dementia of the Alzheimer type:
   1 Memory failure.
   2 Lability of mood.
   3 Apathy.
   4 Depressive or paranoid features.
   5 Parkinsonism.
   6 Parietal lobe syndrome:
      (a) Constructional apraxia – the inability to copy two-dimensional drawings or to construct three-dimensional models.
      (b) Dressing apraxia – the inability to put clothing on properly.
      (c) Ideational apraxia – the inability to voluntarily carry out a sequence of actions.
      (d) Ideomotor apraxia – the inability to copy gestures.
      (e) Anosognosia – denial of the disorder.
      (f) Topographical agnosia – getting lost in familiar surroundings.
      (g) Hemisomatognosia – neglecting one side of the body.
      (h) Autotopagnosia – the inability to recognise, name, or point on command to parts of the body.
      (i) Sensory inattention.
      (j) Cortical sensory loss.
      (k) Astereognosis – the inability to identify objects when placed in the hand.
      (l) Epilepsy.
      (m) Aspects of Gerstmann's syndrome (seen in dominant lobe lesions):
         (i) Right–left disorientation.
         (ii) Finger agnosia – the inability to name fingers.
         (iii) Dyscalculia – difficulty with calculations.
         (iv) Dysgraphia – difficulty in expressing ideas in writing.
   7 Mirror sign – the inability to identify one's own image.
   8 Logoclonia – the monotonous repetition of word particles.
   9 Epilepsy.
   10 Relentless progress of personality and intellectual deterioration.
   11 Aspects of the Kluver–Bucy syndrome:
      (a) Hyperorality.
      (b) Hypersexuality.
      (c) Increased need to touch.
      (d) Placidity.
      (e) Visual agnosia.
      (f) Defects in language and in memory.

II **Alzheimer's disease** – the same disorder as senile dementia of the Alzheimer type, except that it is pre-senile.

III **Multi-infarct dementia:**
  1 Stepwise deterioration in memory.
  2 Perseveration.
  3 Fluctuating cognitive impairment.
  4 Episodes of nocturnal confusion.
  5 Depression.
  6 Hypertension.
  7 Headache.
  8 Dizziness.
  9 Tinnitus.
  10 Scotomata.
  11 Apraxias – the inability to perform voluntary motor acts.
  12 Agnosias – the inability to understand the significance of sensory stimuli.
  13 Aphasia.
  14 Focal neurological deficits.
  15 Personality preservation until late.
  16 Insight intact.

IV **Pick's disease:**
  1 Frontal lobe syndrome:
    (a) Disinhibition.
    (b) Facetious humour, euphoria.
    (c) Irritability, apathy.
    (d) Loss of initiative, decreased intellectual drive.
    (e) Loss of ethical standards, expressive dysphasia.
    (f) Grasp reflex, urinary incontinence.
    (g) Tactlessness, overtalkativeness.
    (h) Reduced verbal fluency, reduced fine motor control.
    (i) Excess in drinking and eating, excess in sexual behaviour.
    (j) Gegenhalten, contralateral spastic paresis.
    (k) Impaired spelling, difficulty in programming and planning behaviour.
  2 Personality deterioration.
  3 Nominal aphasia.
  4 Perseveration.
  5 Amnesia.
  6 Generalised hyperalgesia.

V **Huntington's chorea:**
  1 Insidious onset of choreo-athetoid movements.
  2 Slurring of speech.
  3 Ataxic gait.

4 Intention tremor.
5 Rigidity.
6 Epilepsy.
7 Apathy.
8 Depression.
9 Irritability.
10 Distractibility.
11 Insidious onset of global dementia.
12 Paranoid state.

Differential diagnosis

I   Exclude functional psychiatric disorders:
1   Affective disorders.
2   Schizophrenia.
II   Differentiate dementia from depressive pseudodementia:
Distinguishing features of depressive pseudodementia:
1   Conspicuous subjective difficulty in concentration and remembering but careful clinical testing shows there is no defect of memory function.
2   Psychological symptoms precede the apparent intellectual defects – hence it is important to interview other informants to determine the precise mode of onset.
3   Relatively acute onset.
4   Absence of focal signs.
5   Abreaction or sleep deprivation may clarify the diagnosis.
III   Differentiate dementia from hysterical pseudodementia (including Ganser's syndrome)
Features of Ganser's syndrome:
1   The giving of approximate answers, i.e. answers to simple questions that are plainly wrong but strongly suggest that the correct answer is known.
2   Apparent clouding of consciousness.
3   Dissociative symptoms, e.g. psychogenic amnesia.
4   Conversion symptoms, e.g. ataxia.
5   Pseudohallucinations.

Management

I   Acute organic disorder:
1   Specific measures:
   (a)   The fundamental treatment is directed to the physical cause.
   (b)   In some cases – the effect of appropriate treatment is quite immediate and dramatic, and little more treatment is required, e.g. in the case of hypoglycaemia.
   (c)   In most cases – recovery is more protracted and it is important to observe certain general measures.
2   General measures:
   (a)   The patient should be nursed in a well-lit room, preferably a side ward.
   (b)   Medical and nursing staff should reassure the patient, and explain to him both where he is and what is the purpose of any examination or treatment.
   (c)   The patient should be comfortable, adequately hydrated and in electrolyte balance.
3   Drug treatment:
   (a)   During the daytime:
      (i)   It may be necessary to calm the patient without inducing drowsiness.
      (ii)   The drug choice is haloperidol, which calms without causing drowsiness and postural hypotension, cf. chlorpromazine.
      (iii)   The effective daily dose of haloperidol usually varies from 10 mg to 30 mg.
   (b)   At night:
      (i)   It may be necessary to help the patient sleep.
      (ii)   A suitable drug is a sedative anxiolytic drug (i.e. a benzo-diazepine) which promotes sleep.
   (c)   In the special case of hepatic failure – benzodiazepines may be used during the daytime despite their sedative effects, since they are less likely to precipitate coma, cf. haloperidol (which is the usual drug of choice to calm such patients).
   (d)   In the special case of alcohol withdrawal – chlordiazepoxide is a suitable drug.
II   Chronic organic disorder:
1   Specific measures:
   (a)   If possible the cause should be treated.
   (b)   It is important to detect those cases where treatment can have a marked benefit; for example:
      (i)   Normal pressure hydrocephalus.

(ii)   Hypocalcaemia.
(iii)   Chronic renal failure.
(iv)   Wilson's disease.
(v)   Hypothyroidism.
(vi)   GPI.
(vii)   Space-occupying lesion.
(viii) Vitamin B_{12} deficiency.
(ix)   Alcohol or heavy metal intoxication.

2   General measures:
(a)   The most important consideration – adequate help with self-care and prevention of accidental self-harm.
(b)   Most early cases and many advanced cases – can be managed at home with suitable support, e.g. home helps, district nurses.

3   Drug treatment:
(a)   There are currently several specific drug treatments for dementia – donepezil was the first one to be launched in the UK for the symptomatic treatment of mild or moderate dementia in Alzheimer's disease.
(b)   Other medications can only be used to alleviate certain symptoms:
    (i)   Anxiety – treated with a benzodiazepine or a phenothiazine (e.g. chlorpromazine).
    (ii)   Depressive symptoms – a trial of antidepressant medication is worthwhile even in the presence of dementia.
    NB: TCAs tend to increase confusion in the elderly due to anticholinergic side-effects – therefore SSRIs and SNRIs are the preferred antidepressants.
    (iii) Overactivity/delusions/hallucinations – an antipsychotic may be appropriate, but care is needed to find the optimal dose; in the elderly there are special dangers of hypotension, atropinic effects (such as increasing confusion) and ECG changes – therefore haloperidol is preferred to chlorpromazine in the elderly.
    (iv)   Cognitive impairment – patients with this may be unusually sensitive to antipsychotic drugs; thus, the first doses should be small.

CHAPTER 11

Eating disorders

Anorexia nervosa

Definition

An extreme exaggeration of the widespread habit of dieting. Generally begins with ordinary efforts at dieting in a girl who is somewhat overweight at the time.

Epidemiology

I   **Age:**
    1   Females:
        (a)   Onset usually between ages 16–17.
        (b)   Onset seldom after the age of 30.
    2   Males – onset usually about the age of 12.
II   **Sex:**
    1   More common in females.
    2   The ratio of females to males is about 10:1.
III   **Social class** – more common in upper social classes, i.e. social classes I and II.
IV   **Prevalence rate** – 1% of middle-class adolescent girls.
V   **Incidence** – increasing incidence in recent years, probably due to social pressures. Occurs in 0.5% of adolescent and young adult women.

Clinical features

I   **Main clinical features:**
    1   A body weight more than 25% below the standard weight.
    2   An intense wish to be thin.
    3   Amenorrhoea (in women).

II   Central psychological features:
1   A fear of being fat.
2   Relentless pursuit of a low body weight.
3   The patient has a distorted image of her body – believing herself to be too fat even when severely underweight.
III The pursuit of thinness – this may take several forms:
1   Patients generally eat very little and show a particular avoidance of carbohydrates.
2   Some patients try to achieve this by inducing vomiting, excessive exercise and purging.
3   Some patients have episodes of uncontrollable overeating (binge eating or bulimia):
(a)   After overeating, they feel bloated and may induce vomiting.
(b)   Binges are followed by remorse and intensified efforts to lose weight.
IV   Physical consequences:
1   Clinical features secondary to starvation:
(a)   Sensitivity to cold.
(b)   Constipation.
(c)   Low blood pressure.
(d)   Bradycardia.
(e)   Hypothermia.
(f)   Amenorrhoea (also a primary symptom in a few cases – *see* earlier).
(g)   Leucopenia.
(h)   Abnormalities of water regulation.
(i)   Lanugo hair (hair on trunk).
2   Consequences of vomiting and laxative abuse:
(a)   Hypokalaemia.
(b)   Alkalosis.
(c)   Epilepsy.
(d)   Cardiac arrhythmia.
3   Hormonal abnormalities:
(a)   Elevated hormone levels:
(i)   Growth hormone (GH).
(ii)   Prolactin.
(iii) Cortisol.
(b)   Reduced hormone levels:
(i)   Tri-iodothyronine (T_3).
(ii)   Thyroxine (T_4).
(iii) Oestradiol.
(iv)   Testosterone.
(v)   Follicle-stimulating hormone (FSH).
(vi)   Luteinising hormone (LH).

Aetiology

I   Genetic – 6–10% of female siblings of patients with established anorexia nervosa suffer with the condition.

II   **Hypothalamic dysfunction** – with abnormal control of food intake and reduced sex hormones, which show delayed return on recovery of normal weight.

III   **Social factors:**
  1   High prevalence in upper and middle social classes.
  2   High prevalence in occupational groups particularly concerned with weight, e.g. ballet students.

IV   **Individual psychological causes:**
  1   Disturbance of body image – the three predisposing factors are:
    (a)   Dietary problems in early life.
    (b)   Parents who are preoccupied with food.
    (c)   Family relationships that leave the child without a sense of identity.
  2   Analytical model:
    (a)   Regression to childhood.
    (b)   Fixation at oral (pregenital) level of psychosexual development.
    (c)   Escape from the emotional problems of adolescence.

V   **Causes within the family:**
  1   A specific pattern of relationships can be identified – consisting of:
    (a)   Enmeshment.
    (b)   Overprotectiveness.
    (c)   Rigidity.
    (d)   Lack of conflict resolution.
  2   Development of anorexia nervosa in patient serves to prevent dissension within the family.

Differential diagnosis

I   **Exclude functional psychiatric illnesses:**
  1   Phobic anxiety disorders.
  2   Obsessive compulsive disorders.
  3   Depressive disorders.
  4   Schizophrenia.

II   **Exclude organic disorders:**
  1   Hypopituitarism.
  2   Thyrotoxicosis.
  3   Malabsorption.

    4 Diabetes mellitus.
    5 Neoplasia.
    6 Reticuloses.

Management

I   **Physical** – chlorpromazine and tricyclic antidepressants may be used to promote weight gain. However, the effect is temporary and drug treatment has been superseded by psychological treatment in most centres.

II   **Social** – successful treatment largely depends on making a good relationship with the patient, so that a firm approach is possible. It should be made clear that the maintenance of an adequate weight is an essential first priority.

III   **Psychological:**
    1 Supportive psychotherapy – directed to improving personal relationships and increasing the patient's sense of personal effectiveness.
    2 Family therapy – has been advocated since problems in family relationships are common in anorexia nervosa.
    3 Behavioural therapy – carefully controlled calorie intake:
      (a) A strict regimen of refeeding is carried out.
      (b) Usually behavioural principles are used – i.e. a target weight is set and the patient gains privileges by increasing her weight; e.g. having visitors, trips out of her room.
      (c) Carried out as an in-patient.
    4 Cognitive therapy:
      (a) Aimed at changing the patient's attitude towards eating, and reappraisal of her self-image and life circumstances.
      (b) Usually carried out as an out-patient.

Prognosis

I   **Untreated cases** – the prognosis is very poor.

II   **Treated cases** – the rule of thirds:
    1 One-third – recover fully.
    2 One-third – recover partially.
    3 One-third – little improved or chronically disabled.

III   **Factors associated with a poor prognosis:**
    1 Long illness.
    2 Late age of onset.
    3 Bulimia.

4   Vomiting or purging.
5   Anxiety when eating in the presence of others.
6   Great weight loss.
7   Poor childhood social adjustment.
8   Poor parental relationships.
9   Male sex.
IV **Mortality rate** – 5–10%.

Bulimia nervosa

Definition

Characterised by episodes of uncontrollable overeating (binge eating or bulimia), followed by compensatory behaviours (vomiting, abuse of purgatives).

Epidemiology

Incidence – seen in 1.0–1.5% of women.

Clinical features

Binge eating often of high calorie foods and covertly; bouts of dieting, self-induced vomiting or purgative abuse in an attempt to compensate for binge eating; complications of repeated vomiting – cardiac arrhythmias, renal damage, urinary infections, pitted teeth, epileptic fits, tetany, weakness.

Differences from anorexia nervosa

Patients are usually eager for help; menstrual abnormalities occur in less than half the patients; body weight usually within normal limits.

Similarities to anorexia nervosa

Patients share many psychological features with patients suffering from anorexia nervosa, including an overconcern with body shape and weight; there is often a history of an earlier episode of anorexia nervosa.

Management

I   Physical:
   1   TCAs – produce an immediate reduction in bingeing and vomiting; however, their long-term effects are less pronounced.
   2   SSRIs – fluoxetine is indicated in the treatment of bulimia nervosa (dosage: 60 mg mane; this may be increased to the maximum dosage of 80 mg mane in adults if clinically indicated).

II Psychological:
   1   Group therapy – particularly useful for patients with bulimia nervosa.
   2   Cognitive therapy – also indicated.

CHAPTER 12

Alcohol and drug dependence

Alcohol dependence

Definition

The seven essential elements in the alcohol dependence syndrome are:
I   Subjective awareness of compulsion to drink.
II   Stereotyped pattern of drinking.
III   Increased tolerance to alcohol.
IV   Primacy of drinking over other activities.
V   Repeated withdrawal symptoms.
VI   Relief drinking.
VII   Reinstatement after abstinence.

Epidemiology

I   **Age:**
     1   Heaviest drinkers – men in their late teens or early twenties.
     2   Increasing incidence among adolescents.
II   **Sex:**
     1   More common in males.
     2   Increasing incidence among females.
III **Social class** – lowest prevalence in middle social classes.
IV   **Marital status** – more common in divorced or separated.
V   **Occupation** – certain high-risk occupations, e.g. company directors, doctors, licensed trade.
VI   **Ethnic factors:**
     1   More common in Irish people.
     2   Less common in Jewish people.

Clinical features (psychiatric aspects)

Alcohol-related psychiatric disorders – four groups:

I   **Intoxication phenomena:**
1   Pathological drunkenness – acute psychotic episodes induced by supposedly small amounts of alcohol:
(a)   Individual idiosyncratic reactions to alcohol.
(b)   Usually take the form of explosive outbursts of aggression.
2   Memory blackouts – short-term amnesia:
(a)   Fragmentary lapses up to several hours.
(b)   Frequently reported after heavy drinking.

II   **Withdrawal phenomena:**
1   General withdrawal symptoms:
(a)   Acute tremulousness affecting the hands, legs and trunk ('the shakes').
(b)   Agitation.
(c)   Nausea.
(d)   Retching.
(e)   Sweating.
(f)   Perceptual distortions and hallucinations.
(g)   Convulsions.
2   Delirium tremens – the fully developed withdrawal syndrome:
(a)   Clouding of consciousness.
(b)   Disorientation in time and place.
(c)   Impairment of recent memory.
(d)   Illusions.
(e)   Hallucinations.
(f)   Delusions.
(g)   Agitation and restlessness.
(h)   Fearful affect.
(i)   Prolonged insomnia.
(j)   Tremulous hands.
(k)   Truncal ataxia.
(l)   Autonomic overactivity.

III   **Nutritional or toxic disorders:**
1   **Sustained lack of thiamine:**
(a)   Wernicke's encephalopathy:
(i)   Ophthalmoplegia.
(ii)   Nystagmus.
(iii) Clouding of consciousness with memory disturbance.
(iv)   Ataxia.
(v)   Peripheral neuropathy.

   (b) Korsakoff's psychosis:
     (i)   Impairment of recent memory.
     (ii)   Confabulation.
     (iii)   Retrograde amnesia.
     (iv)   Disorientation.
     (v)   Euphoria.
     (vi)   Apathy.
     (vii) Lack of insight.
     (viii) Ataxia.
     (ix)   Peripheral neuropathy.

2 Alcoholic dementia.

IV **Associated psychiatric disorders:**

1 Alcoholic hallucinosis:
   (a) Auditory hallucinations occurring alone in clear consciousness.
   (b) Voices usually utter insults or threats; may be followed by secondary delusional interpretation.
   (c) The patient is usually distressed by these experiences, appearing anxious and restless.

2 Affective disorder.

3 Personality deterioration.

4 Suicidal behaviour.

5 Sexual problems.

6 Pathological jealousy – the delusion that the marital partner is being unfaithful.

Aetiology

I   **Genetic factors:**

1 Twin studies – show higher concordance rates in MZ than DZ twins.

2 Adoption study – Goodwin (1973) showed significantly higher levels of alcoholism in individuals whose biological parents were known alcoholics and who were adopted in childhood, than in a matched control group.

II **Biochemical factors** – associations reported with abnormalities in:

1 Alcohol metabolising enzymes.

2 Neurotransmitter mechanisms.

III **Learning factors** – children tend to follow their parents' drinking patterns.

IV **Personality factors** – alcohol dependence associated with:

1 Chronic anxiety.

2 Self-indulgent tendencies.

3 A pervading sense of inferiority.

V   **Psychiatric illness** – alcohol dependence occurs in patients with:
1   Anxiety disorders.
2   Phobic anxiety disorders.
3   Affective disorders.
4   Schizophrenia.
5   Organic disorders.
VI **Alcohol consumption in society** – rate of alcohol dependence is related to the general level of alcohol consumption in society.

Management

I   **Physical** – detoxification, i.e. the management of withdrawal of alcohol:
1   Sedation:
    (a) Chlormethiazole (Heminevrin) or chlordiazepoxide (Librium) – sedative drugs generally prescribed to reduce withdrawal symptoms.
    (b) Chlormethiazole may be prescribed in either of two ways:
        (i)   On an as-required basis – i.e. flexibly according to the patient's symptoms.
        (ii) On a reducing regimen basis – i.e. on a fixed six-hourly regimen of gradually decreasing dosage over 6–9 days.
    (c) The patient must stop drinking when taking chlormethiazole – if chlormethiazole is taken in combination with alcohol, each potentiates the CNS depressant action of the other, and overdosage is frequently fatal; thus nowadays chlordiazepoxide is preferred to chlormethiazole.
    (d) Carbamazepine is also indicated in the treatment of acute alcohol withdrawal.
2   Vitamin supplements – to provide B-vitamins: oral multivitamin tablets which contain thiamine, or parenteral preparations if Wernicke's is suspected.
3   Rehydration – to correct any electrolyte imbalance.
4   Glucose – to correct any hypoglycaemia.
5   Antibiotics – to treat any infection.
6   Anticonvulsants – to treat any convulsions, e.g. large doses of chlordiazepoxide may be used.
7   Pharmacological treatments for the maintenance of abstinence after detoxification:
    (a) Disulfiram – an aversive stimulus, inducing nausea in the patient if alcohol is consumed; efficacy limited by problems

with compliance (patients who wish to start drinking again tend to stop the disulfiram to avoid the nausea).

(b) SSRIs – there is some evidence that SSRIs reduce alcohol craving and alcohol consumption in patients with alcohol dependence; however, the results of studies to date have been rather disappointing.

(c) Acamprosate – works on the GABA/glutamate system; licensed in the UK for the maintenance of abstinence.

(d) Naltrexone – an opiate receptor antagonist; licensed in the USA for the maintenance of abstinence.

NB: Both acamprosate and naltrexone are non-addictive, do not interact with alcohol and are associated with relatively few side-effects. Acamprosate and naltrexone may be used in combination to further enhance relapse prevention.

II Social:

1 A goal-orientated treatment plan – these goals should deal with:

(a) The drinking problem:

(i) Total abstinence – a better goal for those aged over 40, who are heavily dependent on alcohol and have incurred physical damage, and who have attempted controlled drinking unsuccessfully.

(ii) Controlled drinking – a feasible goal for those under 40, who are not heavily dependent on alcohol and have not incurred physical damage, and whose problem has been detected early.

(b) Any accompanying problems in:

(i) Health.

(ii) Marriage.

(iii) Job.

(iv) Social adjustment.

2 Other agencies concerned with drinking problems:

(a) Alcoholics Anonymous (AA):

(i) The meetings involve an emotional confession of problems.

(ii) Any patient aiming for abstinence should be recommended to try this organisation.

(b) Hostels:

(i) Provide rehabilitation and counselling; usually abstinence is a condition of residence.

(ii) Intended mainly for homeless problem drinkers.

III Psychological:
1 Psychotherapy:
    (a) Supportive psychotherapy – simple counselling and advice:
        (i)   To educate the patient about the physical, social and psychological complications of alcohol dependence.
        (ii) To help the patient cope with problems in day-to-day living without drinking to excess.
    (b) Group psychotherapy:
        (i)   Aims to enable patients to:
            – Observe their own problems mirrored in other problem drinkers.
            – Work out better ways of coping with their problems.
        (ii) The most widely used treatment for problem drinkers.
        NB: Group psychotherapy will not be helpful while the patient is still actively abusing alcohol.
2 Behavioural therapy:
    (a) Tackles the drinking behaviour itself rather than the underlying psychological problems.
    (b) Includes simple approaches such as self-monitoring, e.g. getting the patient to keep a strict daily log of drinking.
    (c) Often effective.

Prognosis

Factors predicting a good prognosis:
1 First treatment.
2 Motivated.
3 Social stability – in form of:
    (a) A fixed abode.
    (b) Family support.
    (c) Ability to keep a job.
4 Absence of antisocial personality traits – i.e. the ability to:
    (a) Control impulsiveness.
    (b) Defer gratification.
    (c) Form deep emotional relationships.
5 Older.
6 Adequate intelligence.
7 Good insight into nature of the problems.

Drug dependence

Definition

A state, psychic and sometimes also physical, resulting from the interaction between a living organism and a drug, characterised by behavioural and other responses that always include a compulsion to take the drug on a continuous or periodic basis in order to experience its psychic effects and sometimes to avoid the discomfort of its absence. Tolerance may or may not be present.

Epidemiology

I   Age:
  1   Most common in age group 20–30s.
  2   Slight peak in middle age.
II Sex – More common among males.
III Social class:
  1   UK – occurs throughout all social classes.
  2   USA – associated with underprivileged, minority, ethnic groups.

Clinical features

I   Opiates – e.g. heroin:
  1   Both psychic and physical dependence occurs.
  2   Clinical features of chronic opiate dependence:
    (a)   Constipation.
    (b)   Constricted pupils.
    (c)   Chronic malaise.
    (d)   Weakness.
    (e)   Impotence.
    (f)   Tremors.
  3   Withdrawal effects from opiates:
    (a)   Pilo-erection; shivering.
    (b)   Abdominal cramps; diarrhoea.
    (c)   Lacrimation; rhinorrhoea.
    (d)   Dilated pupils; tachycardia.
    (e)   Yawning; intense craving for drug.
    (f)   Agitation; restlessness.

II   **Barbiturates** – e.g. pentobarbitone:
1   Both psychic and physical dependence occurs.
2   Clinical features of barbiturate dependence:
   (a)   Slurred speech.
   (b)   Incoherence.
   (c)   Dullness.
   (d)   Drowsiness.
   (e)   Nystagmus.
   (f)   Depression.
3   Withdrawal effects from barbiturates:
   (a)   Clouding of consciousness; disorientation.
   (b)   Hallucinations; major seizures.
   (c)   Anxiety and restlessness.
   (d)   Pyrexia and tremulousness.
   (e)   Insomnia and hypotension.
   (f)   Nausea; vomiting.
   (g)   Anorexia; twitching.

III   **Hallucinogens** – e.g. lysergic acid diethylamide (LSD):
1   Psychic dependence occurs. Physical dependence does not occur.
2   The mental effects of LSD:
   (a)   Develop during the two hours after LSD consumption; usually last from 8 to 14 hours.
   (b)   Unpredictable and extremely dangerous behaviour; the user sometimes injuring or killing himself through behaving as if he were invulnerable.
   (c)   Mood – acute anxiety, distress or exhilaration.
   (d)   Distortions or intensifications of sensory perception –
      (i)   Synaesthesia – confusion between sensory modalities, e.g. movements are experienced as if heard.
      (ii)   Distortion of the body image – the person sometimes feels that he is outside his own body. These experiences may lead to panic with fears of insanity.

IV   **Amphetamines** – e.g. dexamphetamine:
1   Psychic dependence occurs. A behavioural withdrawal syndrome is recognised.
2   Amphetamine psychosis:
   (a)   Excessive or chronic use of amphetamines, whether taken by mouth or intravenously, induces a paranoid psychosis indistinguishable from acute paranoid schizophrenia.
   (b)   Features:
      (i)   Hostile and dangerously aggressive behaviour.
      (ii)   Prominent persecutory delusions.

(iii) Auditory, visual and tactile hallucinations.

(iv) Clear consciousness.

(c) The condition usually subsides on discontinuing the drug over about a week; however, a few cases continue for months.

(d) It is uncertain whether amphetamine psychosis is a case of schizophrenia provoked by amphetamines, or a true drug-induced psychosis.

V Cannabis – active principle is tetrahydro-cannabinol:

1 Psychic dependence occurs. A behavioural withdrawal syndrome is possible in some.

2 The effects of cannabis:

(a) Exaggerates the pre-existing mood – whether euphoria, depression or anxiety.

(b) Distortion of time and space.

(c) Increased enjoyment of aesthetic experiences.

(d) Intensification of visual perception and visual hallucinations.

(e) Dry mouth; coughing.

(f) Increased appetite; decreased body temperature.

(g) Reddening of the eyes; irritation of the respiratory tract.

3 The adverse effects of cannabis:

(a) A chronic 'amotivation syndrome' in heavy users – blunted motivation, i.e. apathy, decreased drive, lack of ambition.

(b) Psychotic reactions – in patients with a pre-existing psychosis or a vulnerability to psychosis.

(c) Transient 'flashback' phenomena.

VI Cocaine:

1 Psychic dependence occurs. A principally behavioural withdrawal syndrome is also recognised.

2 Formication ('cocaine bugs'):

(a) Characteristic of cocaine dependence.

(b) A bizarre tactile hallucination in which there is a feeling as though insects are crawling under the skin.

VII Benzodiazepines – e.g. lorazepam, diazepam:

1 Both psychic and physical dependence occurs.

2 Clinical features of chronic benzodiazepine dependence:

(a) Unsteadiness of gait.

(b) Dysarthria.

(c) Drowsiness.

(d) Nystagmus.

3 Withdrawal effects from benzodiazepines:

(a) Rebound insomnia; tremor.

(b) Anxiety; restlessness.

(c) Appetite disturbance; weight loss.

(d) Sweating; convulsions.
(e) Confusion; toxic psychosis.
(f) A condition resembling delirium tremens.

Aetiology

I   **Availability of drugs**.
II   **Vulnerable personality**:
   1   People with personality disorder.
   2   People from severely disorganised backgrounds, e.g. a history of childhood unhappiness.
III **Social pressures** – for a young person to take drugs to achieve status, within the immediate peer group.
IV   **Pharmacological mechanisms** – suggestion that tolerance and physical withdrawal effects can be explained by:
   1   An increased neurotransmitter receptor supersensitivity.
   2   Hypertrophy of alternative pathways.
   3   Dysfunction of endorphin metabolism.

Management

I   **Physical**:
   1   'Withdrawal effects from opiates' – two ways of treating:
     (a) Methadone:
       (i)   Given as a mixture in a reducing dosage regimen.
       (ii) Nearly always undertaken as an out-patient.
   NB: To help patients to reduce their methadone from doses of 20 mg (20 ml) or less down to zero, a 21-day lofexidine regimen can be used; blood pressure should be monitored twice a week.
     (b) Symptomatic relief – using chlorpromazine and analgesics.
   2   'Pharmacological treatment for the maintenance of abstinence after detoxification of opiate addicts':
     (a) Initiate naltrexone once the patient has completed detoxification with lofexidine, i.e. after the twenty-first day of the regimen is completed.
     (b) Prescribe half a tablet (25 mg) in the morning on day one.
     (c) From then onwards, prescribe one tablet (50 mg) in the morning for up to six months.
     (d) If the patient continues to abuse opiates while taking naltrexone regularly, they will not experience euphoria.

3 Withdrawal effects from barbiturates:
 (a) Dosage reduction of barbiturate.
 (b) Cover withdrawal symptoms with a benzodiazepine.
 (c) Use anticonvulsants if necessary.
 (d) Nearly always undertaken as an in-patient.
4 Withdrawal effects from benzodiazepines:
 (a) Switch from a short-acting benzodiazepine (e.g. lorazepam) to a long-acting (e.g. diazepam).
 (b) Dosage reduction of benzodiazepine.
 (c) Cover withdrawal symptoms with a sedating antidepressant (e.g. dosulepin 150 mg nocte).
 (d) Undertaken as an out-patient or in-patient.

II **Social**:
'Rehabilitation' – the aim of this is to enable the addict to leave the drug subculture, and develop new social contacts, by way of:
1 The interest and support of a caring person.
2 Accommodation.
3 Work.

III **Psychological**:
'Group psychotherapy':
1 For patients with a vulnerable personality.
2 Used to help patients develop insight into their emotional and personality problems.
3 Group sessions involve intense confrontation with considerable emotional release.

NB: Group psychotherapy will not be helpful while the patient is still actively abusing illicit drugs.

CHAPTER 13
Psychiatric emergencies

Non-fatal deliberate self-harm (DSH)

I **Definition** – a deliberate non-fatal act, whether physical, drug over-dosage or poisoning, done in the knowledge that it was potentially harmful, and in the case of drug overdosage, that the amount taken was excessive.

II **Motives:**
1 The wish to die.
2 'A cry for help' – aimed at changing a seemingly intolerable situation.
3 An attempt to influence other(s) – e.g. seeking to make a relative feel guilty for failing the patient in some way.
4 Escape from emotional distress – the patient seeking immediate relief from his state of mind through temporary oblivion (i.e. unconsciousness).
5 Anger directed at a loved one – and sometimes redirected against the self.
6 Testing the benevolence of 'fate'.

III **Significant predictors of serious suicidal risk in patients following DSH:**
1 Circumstances suggesting high suicidal intent in the DSH act:
    (a) Planning in advance (i.e. premeditated).
    (b) Precautions to avoid discovery.
    (c) Carried out alone.
    (d) No attempts to obtain help afterwards.
    (e) Dangerous or violent method.
    (f) 'Final acts' – e.g. suicide note or making a will.
2 History of previous DSH.
3 Male sex.
4 Older age group (over 45 years old).
5 Psychiatric illness:
    (a) Depressive disorders.
    (b) Alcohol or drug dependence.
    (c) Antisocial personality disorder.

6   Social isolation.

7   Unemployment.

NB: 10% of patients admitted to hospital following DSH commit suicide within 10 years.

The acutely disturbed patient

I   **Aetiology:**
1   Alcohol or drug dependence.
2   Prescribed drugs.
3   Metabolic disturbance.
4   Head injury.
5   Schizophrenia.
6   Mania.
7   Personality disorders.

II **Management** – acutely disturbed behaviour demands immediate action, often before the underlying cause has been determined.
1   Much can be done by providing a calm, reassuring, and consistent environment in which provocation is avoided.
2   A special ward area with an adequate number of experienced staff is much better than the use of heavy medication.
3   However, physical restraint and medication is often needed to bring acutely disturbed behaviour under immediate control:
   (a)   Haloperidol is a better drug than chlorpromazine for this pur- pose, since haloperidol is less sedating, and causes less postural hypotension and fewer anticholinergic side-effects. However, it does have the disadvantage of causing more extrapyramidal side-effects.
   (b)   Up to 18 mg of haloperidol may be given intramuscularly in divided doses for emergency control (up to 30 mg of haloperidol may be given orally in divided doses).
   (c)   If haloperidol alone fails to bring the situation under control, the patient may be given in addition a slow intramuscular injection of 2 mg of lorazepam, if necessary repeated two hours later.
   (d)   If the patient is difficult to persuade to comply with regular oral or intramuscular haloperidol, a short course of injections of zuclopenthixol acetate should be more easily administered; this short-acting injection is more sedative than haloperidol; a maxi- mum of four injections can be given for each course, with a maximum dosage of 150 mg for each injection per 24 hours, and

a maximum dosage of 400 mg for each course of injections. Treatment duration should not exceed two weeks.

(e) IM olanzapine was launched in the UK in 2004, for use in the rapid tranquillisation of acutely disturbed or violent behaviour in patients with schizophrenia or manic episode, when oral therapy is inappropriate:

(i) The recommended initial dose of IM olanzapine is 10 mg.

(ii) A second IM injection, 5–10 mg, may be repeated two hours later.

(iii) The maximum daily dose of IM olanzapine is 20 mg.

(iv) The maximum dose of IM olanzapine is 20 mg in 24 hours on three consecutive days.

(v) Recently it has been recommended that IM lorazepam can only be administered at a minimum of one hour after the administration of IM olanzapine, cf. previously there had been some uncertainty about this as it had been common practice to administer IM lorazepam and IM haloperidol concurrently.

The Mental Health Act (MHA) 1983

I Use:
1 With skill and patience, a sympathetic doctor can often persuade an initially uncooperative patient to accept hospital admission.
2 However, occasionally compulsory hospital admission and detention under the MHA 1983 will be required.
II Indications for compulsory admission and detention under the MHA 1983:
1 The patient must suffer from a mental disorder of a nature and degree which warrants hospital detention for assessment or treatment.
(a) In the interests of his own health or safety.
(b) With a view to the protection of others.
2 There are four categories of mental disorder:
(a) Mental illness.
(b) Mental impairment.
(c) Severe mental impairment.
(d) Psychopathic disorder.
3 The following are not regarded as mental disorders and are therefore excluded from the MHA:
(a) Alcohol or drug dependence.
(b) Promiscuity or immoral conduct.
(c) Sexual deviancy.

III Admission for assessment:
  1 Section 5(2):
     (a) An order for the emergency detention of a patient who is already in hospital as a voluntary patient but wishes to leave.
     (b) It requires a single medical recommendation by the doctor in charge of the case (i.e. the responsible medical officer) or his or her nominated deputy (i.e. the senior house officer in psychiatry).
     (c) The duration of the section is 72 hours.
  2 Section 2:
     (a) An order for the compulsory admission of a patient when informal admission is not appropriate in the circumstances.
     (b) Detention is for assessment, or for assessment followed by medical treatment.
     (c) It requires:
          (i)   Medical recommendation by two doctors, one of whom is a section 12 'approved doctor' (e.g. the specialist registrar or consultant in psychiatry), the other who has preferably previous knowledge of the patient (e.g. the patient's general practitioner).
          (ii) Application by the patient's nearest relative or an approved social worker.
     (d) The duration of the section is 28 days.
  3 Section 4:
     (a) An order for the compulsory detention of a patient in an emergency.
     (b) It should be used only when there is insufficient time to obtain the opinion of a section 12 'approved doctor' who could complete section 2.
     (c) It is usually completed in the patient's home by his or her general practitioner; it is occasionally used in the general hospital casualty department.
     (d) It is expected that a section 4 order will be converted to a section 2 order as soon as possible after the patient has arrived in hospital.
     (e) It requires:
          (i)   Medical recommendation by one doctor, who must have examined the patient within the previous 24 hours; he need not be a section 12 'approved doctor' (e.g. the patient's general practitioner, a senior house officer in psychiatry, a casualty officer).
          (ii) Application by the patient's nearest relative or an approved social worker.
     (f) The duration of the section is 72 hours.

IV **Admission for treatment – Section 3:**
  1 An order for the compulsory admission of a patient for treatment.
  2 It requires:
    (a) Medical recommendation as for section 2. It must specify:
      (i) Which of the four categories of mental disorder the patient is suffering from.
      (ii) Whether any other methods of dealing with the patient are available and, if so, why they are not appropriate.
    (b) Application by the patient's nearest relative or an approved social worker.
  3 The duration of the section is six months.

Index